W9-AHR-263

KNOCKING ON HEAVEN'S DOOR

The Path to a
Better Way of Death

KATY BUTLER

SCRIBNER
New York   London   Toronto   Sydney   New Delhi

Scribner
A Division of Simon & Schuster, Inc.
1230 Avenue of the Americas
New York, NY 10020

Copyright © 2013 by Katherine Anne Butler

All rights reserved, including the right to reproduce this book or portions thereof in any form whatsoever. For information, address Scribner Subsidiary Rights Department, 1230 Avenue of the Americas, New York, NY 10020.

First Scribner hardcover edition September 2013

SCRIBNER and design are registered trademarks of The Gale Group, Inc., used under license by Simon & Schuster, Inc., the publisher of this work.

For information about special discounts for bulk purchases, please contact Simon & Schuster Special Sales at 1-866-506-1949 or business@simonand schuster.com.

The Simon & Schuster Speakers Bureau can bring authors to your live event. For more information or to book an event, contact the Simon & Schuster Speakers Bureau at 1-866-248-3049 or visit our website at www.simonspeak ers.com.

Designed by Jill Putorti

Manufactured in the United States of America

10 9 8 7 6 5 4 3 2 1

Library of Congress Control Number: 2013017659

ISBN 978-1-4516-4197-4
ISBN 978-1-4516-4199-8 (ebook)

32530607433750 ts appear on pages 321–22.

In memory of my parents,
Valerie Joy de la Harpe and Jeffrey Ernest Butler.

In gratitude to Toni Perez-Palma and Alice Teng
and to all caregivers,
paid and unpaid.

I fell
because of wisdom,
but was not destroyed:
through her I dived
into the great sea,
and in those depths
I seized
a wealth bestowing pearl.

I descended like the great iron anchor
men use to steady their ships
in the night on rough seas,
and holding up the bright lamp
that I there received,
I climbed the rope to the boat of understanding.

While in the dark sea,
I slept, and not overwhelmed there,
dreamt: a star blazed in my womb.

I marveled at that light and grasped it,
and brought it up to the sun.

I laid hold on it, and will not let it go.

—MAKEDA, QUEEN OF SHEBA, TRANSLATED BY JANE HIRSHFIELD

CONTENTS

KNOCKING ON
HEAVEN'S DOOR

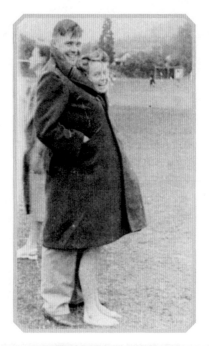

Valerie Joy de la Harpe and Jeffrey Ernest Butler,
Rhodes University, Grahamstown, South Africa, 1946.

PROLOGUE

On an autumn day in 2007, while I was visiting from California, my mother made a request I both dreaded and longed to fulfill. She'd just poured me a cup of tea from her Japanese teapot shaped like a little pumpkin; beyond the kitchen window, two cardinals splashed in her birdbath in the weak Connecticut sunlight. Her white hair was gathered at the nape of her neck, and her voice was low. She put a hand on my arm. "Please help me get your father's pacemaker turned off," she said. I met her eyes, and my heart knocked.

Directly above us, in what was once my parents' shared bedroom, my eighty-five-year-old father, Jeffrey—a retired Wesleyan University professor, stroke-shattered, going blind, and suffering from dementia—lay sleeping. Sewn into a hump of skin and muscle below his right collarbone was the pacemaker that had helped his heart outlive his brain. As small and shiny as a pocket watch, it had kept his heart beating rhythmically for five years. It blocked one path to a natural death.

After tea, I knew, my mother would help my father up from his narrow bed with its mattress encased in waterproof plastic. After taking him to the toilet, she'd change his diaper and lead him tottering to the living room, where he'd pretend to read a book of short stories by Joyce Carol Oates until the book fell into his lap and he stared out the sliding glass window.

I don't like describing what the thousand shocks of late old age were doing to my father—and indirectly to my mother—without telling you first that my parents loved each other and I loved them. That my mother could stain a deck, sew a silk blouse from a photo in *Vogue,* and make coq au vin with her own chicken stock. That her photographs of Wesleyan authors had been published on book jackets, and her paintings of South African fish in an ichthyologists' handbook. That she thought of my father as her best friend.

And that my father never gave up easily on anything.

Born in South Africa's Great Karoo Desert, he was a twenty-one-year-old soldier in the South African Army when he lost his left arm to a German shell in the Italian hills outside Siena. He went on to marry my mother, earn a PhD from Oxford, coach rugby, build floor-to-ceiling bookcases for our living room, and with my two younger brothers as crew, sail his beloved Rhodes 19 on Long Island Sound. When I was a teenager and often at odds with him, he would sometimes wake me chortling lines from *The Rubaiyat of Omar Khayyam* in a high falsetto: "Awake, my little one! Before life's liquor in its cup be dry!" On weekend afternoons, he would put a record on the stereo and strut around the living room conducting invisible orchestras. At night he would stand in our bedroom doorways and say good night to my two brothers and me quoting Horatio's farewell to the dying Hamlet: "May flights of angels sing thee to thy rest!"

Four decades later, in the house where he once chortled and strutted and sometimes thundered, I had to coach him to take off his slippers before he tried to put on his shoes.

My mother put down her teacup. She was eighty-three, as lucid and bright as a sword point, and more elegant in her black jeans and thin cashmere sweater than I could ever hope to be. She put her hand, hard, on my arm. "He is killing me," she said. "He. Is. Ruining. My. Life." Then she crossed her ankles and put her head between her knees, a remedy for near-fainting that she'd clipped from a newspaper column and pinned to the bulletin board behind her. She was taking care of my father for about a hundred hours a week.

I looked at her and thought of Anton Chekhov, the writer and physician who died of tuberculosis in 1904 when he was only forty-four. "Whenever there is someone in a family who has long been ill, and hopelessly ill," he wrote, "there come painful moments when all, timidly, secretly, at the bottom of their hearts long for his death." A century afterward, my mother and I had come to long for the machine in my father's heart to fail.

How we got there is a long story, but here are a few of the bones. On November 13, 2001, when my father was seventy-nine and apparently vigorous, he suffered a devastating stroke. A year later—gravely disabled yet clear-minded enough to know it—he was outfitted with a pacemaker in a moment of hurry and hope. The device kept his heart going while doing nothing to prevent his slide into dementia, incontinence, near-muteness, misery, and helplessness. The burden of his care crushed my mother. In January 2007, when my father no longer understood the purpose of a dinner napkin, I learned that his pacemaker could be turned off painlessly and without surgery, thus opening a door to a relatively peaceful death. It was a death I both feared and desired, as I sat at the kitchen table while my mother raised her head from her knees.

Her words thrummed inside me: *Please help me get your father's pacemaker turned off.* I'd been hoping for months to hear her say something like this, but now that she'd spoken, I was the one with doubts. This was a moral choice for which neither the Anglicanism of my English childhood nor my adopted Buddhism had prepared me. I shook when I imagined watching someone disable his pacemaker—and shook even more when I contemplated trying to explain it to him.

At the same time, I feared that if I did nothing, his doctors would continue to prolong what was left of my father's life until my mother went down with him. My fear was not unfounded: in the 1980s, while working as a reporter for the *San Francisco Chronicle,* I spent six weeks in the intensive care unit of San Francisco General Hospital, watching the erasure of the once-bright line between saving a life and prolonging a dying. I'd never forgotten what I saw.

If my father got pneumonia, once called "the old man's friend" for its promise of an easy death, a doctor might well feel duty-bound to prescribe antibiotics. If he collapsed and my mother called 911, paramedics would do everything they could to revive him as they rushed his gurney toward the emergency room.

With just a little more bad luck, my father might be wheeled into an intensive care unit, where my mother and I—and even my dying father—would become bystanders in a battle, fought over the territory of his body, between the ancient reality of death and the technological imperatives of modern medicine. It was not how we wanted him to die, but our wishes might not mean much. Three-quarters of Americans want to die at home, as their ancestors did, but only a quarter of the elderly currently do. Two-fifths of deaths now take place in a hospital, an institution where only the destitute and the homeless died before the dawn of the twentieth century. Most of us say we don't want to die "plugged into machines," but a fifth of American deaths now take place in intensive care, where ten days of futile flailing can cost as much as $323,000. If my mother and I did not veer from the pathway my father was traveling, he might well draw his last breath in a room stripped of any reminder of home or of the sacred, among doctors and nurses who knew his blood counts and oxygen levels but barely knew his name.

Then again, the hospital might save his life and return him home to suffer yet another final illness. And that I feared almost as much.

I loved my father, even as he was: miserable, damaged, and nearly incommunicado. I loved my mother and wanted her to have at least a chance at a happy widowhood. I felt like my father's executioner, and that I had no choice.

I met my mother's eyes and said yes.

I did not know the road we would travel, only that I'd made a vow. In the six months that followed, I would learn much about the implications of that vow, about the workings of pacemakers and of human hearts, about law and medicine and guilt, about money and morality. I would take on roles I never imagined could be played by a loving daughter. I would watch my father die laboriously with his pacemaker still ticking. After his death, I would not rest until I understood better why the most advanced medical care on earth, which saved my father's life at least once when he was a young man, succeeded at the end mainly in prolonging his suffering.

Researching a magazine article and then this book, I would discover something about the perverse economic incentives within medicine—and the ignorance, fear, and hope within our own family—that promoted maximum treatment. I would contemplate the unintended consequences of medical technology's frighteningly successful war on natural death and its banishment of the "Good Death" our ancestors so prized. Armed with that bitter wisdom, I would support my mother when she reclaimed her moral authority, defied her doctors, refused a potentially life-extending surgery, and faced her own death the old-fashioned way: head-on.

My mother and I often felt like outliers, but I know now that we were not alone. Thanks to a panoply of relatively recent medical advances ranging from antibiotics and vaccines to dialysis, 911 systems, and airport defibrillators, elderly people now survive repeated health crises that once killed them. The "oldest old" are the nation's most rapidly growing age group. But death is wily. Barred from bursting in like an armed man, it wages a war of attrition. Eyesight dims, joints stiffen, heartbeats slow, veins clog, lungs and bowels give out, muscles wither, kidneys weaken, brains shrink. Half of Americans eighty-five or over need help with at least one practical, life-sustaining activity, such as getting dressed or eating breakfast. Nearly a third have some form of dementia, and more develop it with each year of added longevity. The burden of helping them falls heavily on elderly wives and middle-aged daughters, with the remainder provided by sons and husbands, hired caregivers, assisted living complexes, and nursing homes.

Every day across the country, family caregivers find themselves pondering a medical procedure that may save the life—or prevent the dying—of someone beloved and grown frail. When is it time to say "No" to a doctor? To say, "Enough"? The questions surface uneasily in medical journals and chat rooms, in waiting rooms, and in conversations between friends. However comfortingly the questions are phrased, there is no denying that the answers, given or avoided, will shape when and how someone we love meets death. This is a burden not often carried by earlier generations of spouses, sons, and daughters. We are in a labyrinth without a map.

Before I shepherded my parents through to their deaths, I thought that medical overtreatment was mainly an economic problem: a quarter of Medicare's roughly $560 billion in annual outlays covers medical care in the last year of life. After my father's death, I understood the human costs. After my mother's death, I saw that there could be another path.

In our family's case, the first crucial fork in the road appeared six and a half years before my father died, in the fall of 2001. It began with a family crisis, an invitation to a distant daughter to open her heart, and a seemingly minor medical decision: the proposed installation of a pacemaker in the aftermath of a catastrophic stroke.

I

THE STROKE

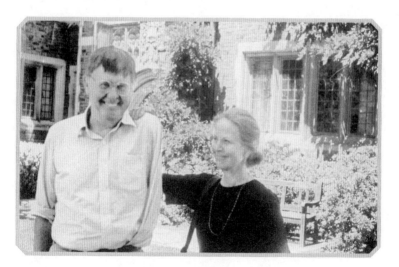

Jeffrey and Valerie Butler, Yale University,
New Haven, Connecticut, 1990.

CHAPTER 1

ALONG CAME A BLACKBIRD

The King was in his counting house,
Counting out his money.
The Queen was in the parlor,
Eating bread and honey.
The Maid was in the garden,
Hanging out the clothes.
Along came a blackbird
And snipped off her nose.

—ENGLISH NURSERY RHYME

Until my parents entered their late seventies, my two younger brothers and I—all of us long settled in California—assumed that they would have robust, vigorous old ages, capped by some brief and vaguely imagined final illness. In my personal fantasy, death would meet my father suddenly after a happy afternoon in my mother's garden, blowing leaves into piles with a rented leaf blower.

Slim and energetic, my parents exercised daily and ate plenty of fish, vegetables, and fruit. Thanks to good doctors and their own healthy habits, they seemed to be among the lucky ones for whom modern medicine, despite its inequities and waste, works quite well. Medicare and supplemental insurance covered their visits to the occasional specialist and to their trusted internist, a lean and bespectacled man in his late forties named Dr. Robert Fales. They didn't have bodies of iron, like some of the graying triathletes I saw at my local swimming pool. But they seemed to be enjoying the thriving, unscathed version of "young old age" that I frequently saw displayed in newspaper features and in the AARP magazine.

They were also stoics and religious agnostics, skeptical of medical overdoing. They'd signed living wills and durable-power-of-attorney documents for health care. My mother, who'd survived cancer and watched friends die of it, even had an underlined copy of the Hemlock Society's *Final Exit* on her bookshelf. They had been, by and large, in control of their lives, and they did not expect to lose control of their deaths.

Then came the stroke, on the afternoon of November 13, 2001.

The day dawned crisp and clear, a Tuesday in late fall, nine days before Thanksgiving and about two months after the attacks on the World Trade Center. My mother had recently turned seventy-seven, my father, seventy-nine. They meditated together for half an hour in the living room and then took their customary brisk two-mile walk down to the Wesleyan campus to pick up the day's *New York Times* from a free rack funded by a wealthy alumnus. The Leonid meteor shower was expected before dawn the following Sunday, and they made plans to get up early to watch the bright rain of shooting stars.

My father helped unload the dishwasher. My mother filled cereal bowls with muesli, All-Bran, soaked prunes, cashews, and apricots. In matching blue-and-white saucers she placed handfuls of vitamins recommended by the Center for Science in the Public Interest, along with a diuretic for her moderately high blood pressure and a generic pill for his enlarged prostate. After breakfast, she headed upstairs to make their twin beds in the master bedroom; they no longer shared a bed because of my father's snoring. My father went into the second upstairs bathroom—the one my two brothers and I shared when we were younger—and, for the last time in his life, took a shower on his own and shaved.

A few hours later, I awoke in the flats of Mill Valley, California, in the redwood house I'd just begun to share with my partner, Brian Donohue, whom I met in a salsa class a year before. In my makeshift study there—formerly his oldest son's bedroom, with a *Fight Club* poster still on the wall—I revised an article I'd written for *Tricycle,* a Buddhist quarterly. I was fifty-two, my parents' oldest child and their only daughter.

My father had lunch at the Wesleyan faculty club, listened to a former colleague lecture on Cuba, drove home, and took a nap. He was taking a break from revising the book that had consumed nearly twenty years of his life, a fine-grained study of racial inequity and apartheid in Cradock, the South African desert town where he was born. His editors at the University of Virginia Press had asked for substantial cuts, and my mother believed that "the bloody book" was ruining his retirement; she wanted him to permanently abandon it.

At a quarter to four, in the kitchen of their open, sun-filled, midcentury modern house on a grassy slope above Middletown, Connecticut, my father put on the kettle for tea and fell to the floor making burbling sounds. Somewhere in his heart, in an aged, stiffened, and partly clogged artery, a yellowish-white clump of fatty cells and microscopic chalky debris about the size of a baby aspirin had worked its way loose from a vessel wall. Carried by the tides of his pumping blood, it drifted upward to the left side of his neck, plugged a secondary branch of his carotid artery, and deprived whole neighborhoods of his brain of blood and oxygen. Among the neighborhoods that suffered most was Broca's area, beneath the thin bone of his left temple, where specialized chains of cells help us find words and speak sentences. Another damaged area lay on the left side of his motor cortex, a strip of brain cells that arches over the top of the skull like a hair band, from ear to ear, and is responsible for physical movement. My father was paralyzed on his right side; he couldn't get up from the floor.

He was still burbling there when my mother came downstairs, let out a cry, and called 911. By the time his ambulance arrived at the doors of the emergency room of Middlesex Memorial, the town's excellent nonprofit hospital, whole swaths of the father I'd known for half a century were gone. The machinery of advanced lifesaving swung into motion: he was scanned and tested and moved rapidly into an intermediate intensive care unit, where he was given an oxygen tube and, because he could not swallow, a temporary feeding tube as well. About seven hundred thousand Americans have strokes each year. It is a predictable hazard of late old age: people over seventy-five are ten times more likely to have one than those in their late fifties. One of my parents' closest neighbors, the historian William Manchester, had recently had two of them. Nevertheless, my father's stroke came as a complete surprise to us.

There had been omens over the prior year, had any of us wanted to see them. A CAT scan, taken when my father was complaining of terrible headaches whose origins were never pinpointed, revealed what a radiologist called "mild generalized brain atrophy"—that is, shrinkage—"consistent with the patient's age." On a vacation I took with my parents to Jefferson's Monticello, my father came back from a meeting with his book editor in Charlottesville strangely thrown by the prospect of revising his footnotes. Finally, a gastroenterologist, alarmed by a slow heartbeat detected during a routine colonoscopy, referred my father to a cardiologist to be assessed for a pacemaker. Before the cardiac tests could be completed, however, the stroke hit, taking with it all our illusions of my father's immortality.

My mother did not call me until she got back from the hospital hours later. As soon as I heard her strangled, defenseless cry, before I could even decipher her words, something visceral and hot rose up in me, pulling my heart and guts toward Middletown. "Katy! Jeff's had a stroke," she wept, and then took a breath and said, "Don't come." I don't think I'd ever heard her say, "I need you," just as I'd rarely said those words to her since I was a lonesome girl of sixteen and she dropped me off at boarding school.

"What should I do?" I asked Brian after hanging up. He was fifty-one then, bear-like and gentle, with a beautiful singing and speaking voice. He sold operating-room tables and lights for a living, and loved to play guitar and recite poems learned by heart. "Don't listen to her," he said calmly, holding me. He grew up in a warm, extended Irish-American family in a duplex in Queens still occupied by his widowed and arthritic eighty-seven-year-old father, who got by with help from a daily housekeeper and support from neighbors and cousins.

"Find a flight," Brian said, "and just tell her when your plane is landing."

My two brothers, when I called them, made no move to drop everything and go. Neither had been as close to my father as I was in childhood; it was almost as if we'd grown up in different families. My brother Michael was forty-eight. Lean, empathic, a natural mimic, and a wonderful guest at a dinner party, he had a genius for living elegantly on next to nothing and was studying improvisational theater at a community college near me in Northern California. His relationship with our parents had long been difficult. Much to their distress, he faded in and out of their lives like a distant lighthouse, often going for months without phoning and years without visiting. As soon as he was sure our father wasn't actively dying, he showed no interest in flying east.

I reached Jonathan, my ebullient youngest brother, in the garage of his shared, rented house on Lake Elsinore in the Southern California desert. He was living on his tax refund, taking a break from driving eighteen-wheelers across the country, and rebuilding the engine of his own truck, a secondhand 1986 Ford F-150. Forty-six, bright, and dyslexic like our mother, with no education beyond high school, he was intensely practical, the kind of person you'd want next to you in an earthquake or a hurricane. He could embroider an American flag on the back of a Levi's jacket, pilot a loaded semi through Grapevine Canyon in the Tehachapi Mountains, and navigate a sailboat along the rocky Maine coast. But he lived from paycheck to paycheck and had long felt that our father neglected him as a child, dismissed him as an academic failure, and didn't value his mechanical skills or his seventeen years of hard-won sobriety. In any case, this wasn't Jonathan's kind of natural disaster. "I've seen it over and over," he would tell me years later, when I asked why he hadn't come. "Everyone jumps on an airplane, they go to the emergency room, and they stand there together for hours drinking shitty coffee out of the vending machine. They do it out of guilt, they become a burden, and they accomplish nothing."

And so it turned out that only my mother and I sat on the empty second bed in my father's room at Middlesex Memorial Community Hospital in Middletown, facing the wreckage of a man whom we desperately loved and whose future we could not know. Stripped of his spotless white shirt and nice tweed jacket, his commanding Oxford accent, his height and apparent confidence, he was in a wheelchair, catheterized and naked beneath a pale hospital gown, a member of the classless fraternity of the stricken.

An occupational therapist bent up his right arm—his only arm—and asked him to keep it raised. She watched it flop down. She pointed to her watch and asked my father to name it. What came out of his mouth were stutters. As the therapist finished up her notes, she suggested my dad practice pursing his lips and blowing, so that someday he could maneuver a breath-controlled motorized wheelchair.

My father pursed his lips.

Thank God, I thought. He understands her.

And Oh God, I thought. A breath-controlled wheelchair.

His lips made a circle and he puffed out his cheeks and blew. It was a gesture I remembered from fifty years before.

I was a child of three. I sat on his lap in our garret apartment in Oxford, England, watching in wonderment as he gravely drew on his pipe, filled his cheeks, pursed his lips, snapped his jaw, and puffed out rings of blue-white smoke: a round one, then an oval, then a wavering square that expanded and broke apart as it rose into the air. I thought he was a wizard. I was then his only child.

My father was a student at Oxford then. We lived on what he earned teaching at night school and on the disabled veterans' pension that came every month in a windowed envelope stamped with the crest of the South African government. Food was rationed. Clothing was rationed. Everyone in England was in the same boat.

One day he and my mother drove a borrowed car to a small brick and stone row house on Thorncliffe Road in North Oxford, our new home. Out the kitchen window, beyond the wringer washer, was a flagstone path, a peony bush, and a ladder leaning against an apple tree. A strange, feathery white mold grew in the cellar. A black dray horse named Flower clopped up the street twice a week, his cart full of cabbages and leeks. Milk was left on the doorstep at dawn under red clay pots, the bottles lidded with silver foil and collared white with cream.

In the depths of winter there were paisleys of ice painted in whorls on the inside of our windows. I would watch my father leave for his university classes with his breath rising like mist from the street, his short black undergraduate's gown flapping like bat wings as he grasped the handles of his bicycle near the pivot-point with his one hand, mounted and wobbled, regained his balance, and rode away.

One evening, he was standing just inside the kitchen doorway when all the plaster fell down from the ceiling. He had chips of white in his hair. My mother turned to him, eyes gleaming, and said, "It's coming, it's coming." I was sent off to spend the night with my best friend. The next morning, the plaster was swept up and the ceiling lath was showing. The midwives from the National Health Service were packing their black bags. My father brought me up to the big bedroom to see my new brother, Michael. But I remember only the gleam of the electric heater and my mother lying on a rubber sheet with her blond hair sweaty and loose on the pillow. When Michael was two and still in diapers, the midwives came again, and then I had two brothers. I wished they would both disappear.

It was my father, not my mother, who taught me how to take a bath. First he'd turn on the cold water, for safety, then the hot. He showed me how to soap up my washcloth and wipe my nose and ears. To rinse. To stand with the right foot up on the rim of the tub and scrub between my toes. To sit down and soap my armpits and the clefts of my body.

He told me stories about growing up in a desert so dry and empty that a farmer could descry a neighbor coming on horseback from forty miles away by the column of dust he kicked up. He told me about shooting a coiled, hissing, poisonous snake called a puff adder in the rocky foothills, about putting a loud but harmless homemade bomb on the Cradock railroad tracks, about breaking both arms slipping from a homemade trapeze that his father, who ran the town's struggling daily newspaper, hung from a backyard pear tree.

He bought me *Oliver Twist* and the African adventure novels of H. Rider Haggard, and *Jock of the Bushveld,* about a hunting dog and his master who rode ox wagons in the wild South African interior between the Cape of Good Hope and the gold and diamond camps.

He taught me to read when I was four. He was sure I was the brightest little girl in Oxford. I wanted to make him proud.

He gave me the Christmas presents he'd yearned for as the youngest of five children growing up in the Depression: a Lionel train set, a working model steam engine, and a tiny airplane with a high-pitched motor that flew on a wire The love he showed me settled deep in my heart and marrow, in a place far below thought.

In the evenings we would lie on the carpet before the fire, and I would touch the scars on his cheek, his calf, the back of his hand—his body a map that I loved to make him explain.

"Tell me the story," I'd say, "of how you lost your arm."

During the Second World War in Italy, he'd volunteered for armed reconnaissance, seeking out and destroying small pockets of retreating Germans as the Allies fought their way up the Italian boot. A shell burst over his foxhole in the mountains near Siena. Shrapnel hit his head and both hands, and his left arm was shredded. After he came to—and here my father would raise his one hand, his fingers splayed out in the firelight—the first thing he did was reach for his gun.

"It was then," he would say, "that I knew I was a man."

In a field hospital set up in a farmhouse with a red canvas

cross on the roof, my father's left arm turned black with gan-
grene. The doctors weren't sure he'd live through the night. A
mortar hit the roof. Before he passed out, a shower of white
dust fell from the rafters onto his face.

Doctors amputated his left arm at the shoulder and saved
his life.

To fight the infections coursing through his bloodstream, they
shot him full of a miraculous new drug first discovered in London
in the 1920s but not widely deployed until the Second World
War, when American and British scientists and military person-
nel teamed up to manufacture it on a mass scale, using a hardy
"mother" mold discovered on a rotting melon in a market in Peoria, Illinois. I never heard my father thank God for his miraculous
survival. He thanked Sir Alexander Fleming and penicillin.

Now we were thousands of miles and decades away from South
Africa, England, and Italy. Medical advances such as those that
saved him as a twenty-one-year-old had once again been deployed.
But how far could miracles reach? The man who taught me how
to take a bath would never again take one on his own. The man
who taught me to revel in words and stories could not speak.

An orderly walked into the room: a short, squat man in his
fifties with longish hair, a belly pushing against his green V-neck
hospital scrubs, and a blurred blue anchor on his right bicep. He
carried a can of foam, a plastic bowl half-full of warm water, a
disposable razor, and a hand towel. After nodding to my mother
and me, he sat down on a plastic chair, perpendicular to my
father's wheelchair, and looked at his face.

He did not banter, talk down, or coo. He pressed white
lather into the palm of one hand and softly daubed my father's
ruddy cheek. He held my father's chin and stroked his razor up
that cheek with tenderness. He took all the time in the world.

roo and she the baby. They had not yet bickered and shouted and taken each other for granted and quietly contemplated divorce and seen each other through disappointments and softened and reconciled. They were laughing. My mother was barefoot. She had just won a footrace, and it was starting to rain.

The orderly dipped his razor into the water.

In the early 1970s, after graduating from Wesleyan, I gave up my shared rented apartment and drove cross-country to California, part of the great baby-boom diaspora from small towns to cities on the coasts. I was doing what generations of middle-class children had done since the Industrial Revolution: going off to seek my fortune, forgetting that blood is thicker than water, and not looking back. By then, my father and I had long been estranged, our easy early intimacy lost to years of fights over my undone homework and messy bedroom and his bad temper and expectations, never met, that I get straight As.

Desperate to become a writer, I landed in San Francisco chasing the success I secretly hoped would make him proud and that I was sure would elude me as long as I remained within the force field of his baleful doomsaying. I wrote for an alternative weekly and then for the *San Francisco Chronicle*, the big morning daily. Twelve years later I quit to freelance for magazines. I married and divorced. I made my own life. I visited my parents once a year, and sometimes not even that often.

Of course we kept in touch. When I was still in my twenties, my father wrote me a remorseful letter acknowledging that not long after we came to America, he'd "become insanely ambitious for you and let all the love go out of the relationship." Our edges softened. He lent me half the down payment for my first San Francisco house. On my birthdays, he would write me tender, formal, almost Victorian letters. Several times a year, I would

He paid close attention to what he was doing and investe
moment, the room, with a presence I can only call sacred.

The hospital may well have saved my father's life with
sands of dollars' worth of oxygen, liquid nourishment, s
X-rays, intravenous lines, feeding tubes, barium-swallowing
catheters, and other sophisticated treatments and diagnostic

Now I watched someone tenderly touch him.

Fearful of the notorious impersonality of modern hosp
I'd taped family photographs above my father's bed to n
sure nurses knew we cared what happened to him. My S
African mother told everyone who entered the room that
husband lost his arm in the Second World War—"fighting
Demaacracy," she'd say ironically, in a broad American acc
as she was fighting for his dignity now. But the orderly did
need family photographs or a war history to treat my father v
reverence. We were in an oasis of caring, everything the mod
hospital aspires to be and rarely is. And I was learning, fro
fat man with a tattoo whose name I didn't know, how to love
helpless, broken, and infinitely slowly dying father.

My mother twisted her hands in her lap and sat, unchar
teristically quiet. Among the photographs I'd stuck above
bed was a family favorite, taken in 1946, of her and my fatl
on a playing field at Rhodes University in South Africa's Easte
Cape. She was twenty-two in the photograph, and he was twen
four. It was taken only a few months before they walked out
the Grahamstown church together, all dressed up and grinnir
with her white veil thrown back and his black hair flecked wi
confetti and rice. Two years before they sailed away to Englar
with me in a bassinet, and more than a decade before they saile
the Atlantic, this time towing three young kids, relying mainly o
each other and their own guts to build a successful, even elegan
American émigré life. In the photo, they were both buttoned int
my father's army overcoat, as though he were the mother kanga

send him articles I'd written, like a teenager still yearning for Daddy's approval.

Every March, after teaching a writing workshop in Washington, DC, I would take the Amtrak Acela north and be picked up by my parents in New Haven. When it was warm enough, my father and I would linger over breakfast on the deck beneath a lattice of green unfurling Dutchman's Pipe vines, parrying happily over something in that morning's *New York Times* while my mother washed the dishes. We'd duck and dart behind walls of words. Often I wasn't sure what he really thought.

The rest of the time, I was comfortable loving my parents from a distance.

The orderly asked my father to turn his cheek.

As my father turned his head, his eyes caught the glossy stitching of the red chenille sweater I was wearing, bought at a secondhand store. It was the kind of visual detail he'd rarely noticed when his powerful, professorial left brain was intact.

The stroke had stripped away our shared vocabulary of oblique love along with his capacity to speak. In the years to come, I would express my love for him less in words than in acts. And as my father cast off the husks of his old life, I found myself overwhelmed by a deep underwater love rising from depths I was just beginning to plumb.

Finding the right word for one of the first times since the stroke, he said, "Beautiful."

Later that day, or early the next—I don't remember—the hospital's "discharge planner" told us that my father had to be transferred to a center for neurological rehabilitation at once. Only later would I understand the rush: the hospital was losing money on him with every passing day. Out of $20,228 in services billed, Medicare would reimburse Middlesex Memorial only $6,559, a lump sum based on the severity of my father's stroke diagnosis. (Losses are absorbed by charitable donations and, in what is known as cost-shifting, revenue from more profitable departments and better-insured patients.) This lump-sum system, known as the DRG (for diagnosis-related group), was instituted in the 1980s during a period of rapid medical inflation to force hospitals to control costs. But it also incentivized rapid discharges, turned patients into items on conveyor belts, and eroded the hospital's traditional role as a place for nursing, convalescence, and healing.

I drove my mother to the closest place with an available bed, a high-rise rehab center in the poor city of New Britain. In a panicked rush, she accepted it—the first but not the last snap decision she would make in her new role as my father's medical guardian. We followed my father's ambulance there and nervously watched the orderlies unload him. I was terrified he'd somehow shatter, like a cracked glass.

The place had been recommended by Dr. Fales, my parents' internist. The TV blared in the dayroom all day, there was no access to the natural world, and my father, who was spontaneously recovering some speech, strung together enough words to tell my mother vehemently, "Get me the *hell* out of here." She and I drove south to Gaylord Rehabilitation Institute in rural Wallingford, and my hopes lifted when we toured its leafy campus, with its Disney-like indoor "Main Street" where the brain-damaged could practice buying apples or toothpaste or simply walking in a straightish line holding onto a rail. In 1989, six months of intense rehabilitation at Gaylord had helped a young Salomon Brothers investment banker, whom the newspapers called the Central Park Jogger, learn to walk and speak again after her skull was bashed in with a brick.

Perhaps my father, too, could be fixed.

I was thinking in confused ways then. First I'd fantasize about sending for Berlitz language-immersion tapes and drilling my father until he could speak fluently and fully understand English again. Then I'd hope he'd have another stroke and die. The one scenario I didn't consider was the likely one, spelled out for us in a brochure we were given: stroke victims tend to improve rapidly for about a year and then the gains taper off. They live, on average, with varying degrees of disability, for another seven.

Gaylord had no empty bed.

I sprang into action like the reporter I was, like the man my father had been, and like the substitute husband my mother needed. I spun her Rolodex. I negotiated with a social worker at the New Britain rehab. My mother called a friend whose former husband was on the Gaylord board and whose daughter was a doctor. I called the daughter. We begged. We waited. I said we'd cover whatever charges Medicare wouldn't pay. It gave us something to do. We thought we were making a difference. It was just about the only way we could show our love.

Perhaps because of our efforts, or perhaps just by luck, a bed opened up at Gaylord. Relieved that things seemed on the way to being settled, at least for the moment, I booked my return flight west. A close friend of my mother's promised to help ensure that my father's transfer to Gaylord went smoothly, and one of my father's former colleagues drove me to the airport.

Within hours my plane was descending over San Francisco Bay, the dark silhouette moving across the steely waters in the late afternoon light. At its southern edge, the vast Cargill salt evaporation ponds welcomed me home—as they often would over the next eight years—their algae-tinted yellows, oranges, and blue-greens patched together as oddly and beautifully as a Gee's Bend sharecropper's quilt. Behind me in Connecticut lay my father, wounded more grievously than I knew, and a mother who had never balanced a checkbook.

The seat-belt sign blinked off.

I did not think of my father as dying. I did not even think of him as "in decline." I thought of him as staggering from a terrible, unexpected blow.

Brian would meet me at the gate. I'd pick up my life where I'd left it. I'd deploy the skills I'd acquired as a journalist to help my formidable parents, whom I considered embodiments of ingenuity and the can-do spirit. Given their guts, my research, and their doctors' expertise, I dimly hoped things would come out right.

I was like the drunk who searches for his keys in front of the streetlamp because the light is better there, even though he dropped them up the street. The kaleidoscope that had been our family's life—with its familiar roles and hierarchies, its intricate alliances, secret wounds, loves, and memories—had shifted in ways I didn't yet understand. What once looked like a jeweled snowflake was now a dark flower. We came from a long line of doers and strivers, and from now on, doing and striving would carry us only so far.

It would take me more than a year to realize that my father had walked through the invisible gate that separates the autumn of healthy old age from the hidden winter of prolonged and attenuated dying. The time for fixing was over. The glass was already broken. The landscape had changed.

CHAPTER 2

A YEAR OF GRACE

On a midsummer morning eight months after the stroke, my parents and I sat meditating in their spare, impeccable living room on Pine Street in Middletown. The sliding glass doors opened onto the deck, and the last of the previous night's cool air seeped through the screens. My privacy-mad mother had sited the house so carefully that no neighbor's dwelling was visible—only the Dutchman's Pipes that enclosed the deck in a cutwork of translucent green. Beyond that lay a long, sloping lawn, the birch trees she'd planted forty years earlier, and the rolling hills of the Connecticut River Valley, glimpsed through hedges and clumps of trees.

The knobs of my sitting bones pressed onto my meditation bench, and my shins rested on the fleece of the white Flokati rug. My father sat flaccidly on the couch, his only hand curled upward in his lap, and his right shoulder slumped. In out-of-character red suspenders and a neatly trimmed beard, he looked more like a retired hippie watchmaker than the dignified, clean-shaven academic he'd once been. My mother had stripped him of most of the markers of adult life: his belt, keys, wallet, Wesleyan ID, and credit cards—even, for reasons I couldn't fathom, his stainless-steel watch on its expandable metal band. She was sitting on her own bench in dark yoga clothes, her spine fiercely erect, her lovely white hair falling over her shoulders.

I cast my eyes down. My mind repeated phrases I'd learned more than a decade earlier from Thich Nhat Hanh, my Vietnamese Zen teacher: *I breathe in, making my whole body calm and at peace. I breathe out, making my whole body calm and at peace.* My shoulders let go. The dial of the kitchen timer at my knee, set for twenty minutes, turned a little closer to zero.

The room was so clean and orderly and the views so tranquil that I felt as though I were at a retreat center. It was nothing like my chaotic life in California.

I breathe in . . .

Not long after I moved west, I learned not to visit my parents more than once a year or to stay for more than three days in a row. After the first excited, intimate babble of catching up, I could count on my mother exploding over something, or a series of somethings, that I considered trivial: not hanging my towel up to dry each day in the basement; wanting an extra blanket; eating too much expensive Manchego cheese; leaving three grains of rice in the dish drain; using too much heat, hot water, electricity, paper towels, or dish soap.

Sometimes I was the one to explode over things my mother found equally trivial: entering my bedroom without knocking; hinting that I should lose or gain five pounds, wear more neutral colors, or stop tinting my hair brown when it would look so marvelous gray. My father, in his vital, prestroke days, would croon, "Dooon't Es-ca-late!" over our rising voices, my mother would call me selfish or oversensitive, and I'd race upstairs to book an earlier flight home, hating her and craving her love at the same time.

I breathe out . . .

In many ways, she and I were mirror images, both in love with the same preoccupied and now severely damaged man, each brilliant in realms where the other could barely cope. She couldn't spell, had no idea how much they had saved, made any room she entered more beautiful, and ran her house with the precision of a fine Swiss watch. I left something askew everywhere I went, paid my own mortgage, and had never been supported by a man or taken care of a sentient being more complex than a ficus tree. She wanted a different daughter—one more feminine, graceful, and considerate. I wanted a mother—warm, tolerant, nurturing—that she'd never been nor could be.

And there I was, sitting quietly in their living room, back in their house on Pine Street for the third time in eight months, for yet another open-ended stay.

My father coughed and shifted on the couch. A fly buzzed, hit the screen of the sliding door, and stopped. It shifted first a front leg, then a back. I consciously let my shoulders go.

My mother rose on her haunches, stripped off her flip-flop, and thwacked at the screen. *What's wrong with her? Can't she sit still for twenty minutes!*

Right Speech is an integral part of Buddha's noble eightfold path. I composed tactful words in my head: *Ma, I was hoping. . . .* She thwacked and thwacked. The fly leaped. I rose, giggling, put a soft hand on her shoulder, and whispered my request that she wait till we'd finished meditating She smiled back, let go of her flip-flop, and sat back down. Ten minutes later, the timer went off with a ding, and the three of us went into the kitchen for breakfast. That was all.

It was a small thing, perhaps—that fight we didn't have. But later, when I looked back on our first year in the long corridor of my father's dying, I would treasure that moment of grace. Was it our daily meditation, my mother's forbearance, my attempts to practice my latest self-help technique, called Nonviolent Communication? Our stunned humility? The fact that my parents needed me? All I know is that during that first year, carried in part by gimcrack hopes, we rose above our ordinary selves. Our hearts opened. We were on a honeymoon. And we needed to be.

I did not believe in God then, and I don't now. But the closest I can come to explaining what happened during that year of grace is to describe a Christian poster I once saw and thought at the time was sentimental, of footprints along the damp sand of a beach. The script along the bottom read, "During your times of trial and suffering, when you saw only one set of footprints, it was then that I carried you."

That year of grace began in a state of stunned despair. My father came home after just three weeks at Gaylord Rehabilitation Institute, far from dead and far from fixed. My mother told me that he could not fasten a belt or put on a shirt, and he walked with his right foot dragging. At night he wet his bed. On the phone to me, his speech was a flurry of blithers and stutters, of words sought and missed, of phrases begun and halted in midair, followed by a pause, a garbled "I must go," and a sudden hang up. Then, once in a while, he would come out with a complete sentence, clear as a bell.

One day he said to my mother, "I don't know who I am any more."

A Medicare-funded speech therapist named Angela came to the house and helped him learn to write again and to do simple arithmetic. She told my mother not to give up, that my father was still in there, intact, just unable to speak clearly. "*Every day* sees improvement for Jeff," my mother wrote cheerfully to my father's three elderly sisters in South Africa. "In some ways he is ahead of the game, having lived with his one arm since he was twenty-one. So you see I have reason to feel optimistic."

On the phone with my brothers and me that winter, she cried. She loved my father. She'd vowed to be with him in sickness and in health, she told us—and who was she to think they'd escape the sickness part? He'd taken care of her for fifty years, and now it was her turn. But in ways we were only beginning to fathom, my father was no longer her husband, and she was no longer his wife.

His stroke devastated two lives. The day before it, my mother was a talented amateur artist and photographer, a woman of intimidating energy, and a spectacular homemaker. She sewed almost all her own clothes and was halfway through knitting a sweater out of pale blue chenille ribbon, mimicking one she'd seen in an Eileen Fisher catalog. She took hikes with women she liked, cooked wonderful dinners for my father and their friends, went to the bookstore and the library, read voraciously, nagged and happily bantered with my father, cleaned and gardened, and practiced Japanese calligraphy in her spare time.

After the stroke, she cared for my father the way she'd cared for my brothers and me when we were three or four. In the morning, she helped him up from bed, brushed his teeth, gave him a shower, laid out his clothes, tucked a thick incontinence pad in his underwear, and helped him put on his shirt, pants, socks, and shoes. She fastened his belt, buttoned his buttons, cut his toenails, put in his hearing aids, put on his jacket, brushed his hair, and then took him to appointments, often three or more in a single week, with his neurologist, internist, physical therapist, dentist, or eye doctor. She helped him get up and down when he took a nap. She tried to wait patiently when he couldn't find a word. When he wanted to go to the bathroom, she helped him take down his pants and wiped his bottom. She even took him grocery shopping—she did not feel comfortable leaving him alone. At night, she repeated the process in reverse, starting with his hearing aids, and then collapsed into a single bed in the former guest room, under a poster of the artist Frida Kahlo. Sometimes at night she would get up two or three times to change his wet sheets.

She no longer went to yoga classes or to the bookstore or invited people to dinner, and rarely walked alone or with her friends. In time, most dinner invitations from others stopped as well. Her sewing machine was silent. Her half-finished ribbon sweater sat in her sewing basket for six years. At seventy-seven, she had become one of twenty-nine million unpaid, politically powerless, and culturally invisible family caregivers—9 percent of the U.S. population—who help take care of someone over seventy-four.

On a routine visit to her internist, Dr. Fales, two months after the stroke, she burst into tears. "Even though she is a rather stoic individual," Dr. Fales would write in his clinical notes, "She seems to be beside herself because she can simply not cope with trying to handle Mr. Butler's physical condition and all of the financial affairs which have now fallen in her lap. She does have a reliable daughter to help her through this difficult time."

Dr. Fales spent thirty minutes with her—twice the allotted time. "I bonded with your parents, and you don't bond with everybody," he would later tell me. "It's easier to understand someone if they just tell it like it is from their heart and their soul."

He gave her a prescription for Ambien, a sleeping pill. But she needed more than a pill and a so-called reliable daughter three thousand miles away. She needed a support team—a social worker, a visiting nurse, and hired caregivers to give her respite. Our whole family, in fact, could have used help: with the confused, muffled grief we felt about having a paterfamilias who was no longer in charge; with the disappointment I felt about my brothers being AWOL; with medical decisions we did not even know we would need to make; and with our disowned, premonitory sadness about the unnameable losses yet to come. Had my father been diagnosed with a reliably fatal disease such as pancreatic cancer, we would have gotten such help from a Medicare-funded hospice team. But the Medicare hospice benefit is reserved for unambiguous dying. It covers only those who give up all hope of cure and are certified by a doctor to have less than six months to live. The requirements are so draconian—and doctors and some families so overoptimistic about the patients' survival chances—that half of those who enter hospice get care for no more than their last eighteen days of life.

If my father had died of his stroke, we would have had a big funeral. Covered dishes would have appeared on the doorstep and condolence letters in the mail. Kind friends would have taken my mother to dinner, and single women would have befriended her, acknowledging her new social identity, her widowhood. Former colleagues would have known more or less what to do and say. But there is no public ceremony to commemorate a stroke that blasts your brain utterly, and no common word to describe the ambiguous state of a wife who has lost her husband and become his nurse.

I would later read, in a remarkable caregiver's manual by Dr. Dennis McCullough called *My Mother, Your Mother,* that this was the moment for me to fly in, capitalize on the outpouring of phone calls that followed the stroke, and marshal concerned friends and neighbors to help in specific ways. But I was busy earning a living, and my proud, self-reliant parents had not invited me to manage their lives. My mother, a solitary being and a perfectionist, was in some ways her own worst enemy. She doubled down and did more of what she already did well: working tirelessly, frugally, and efficiently, and asking for nothing. When a younger female history professor she barely knew

offered to come sit with my father and give her respite, she
didn't follow up. When visiting home-health aides, funded for
a few hours a week by Medicare, showed up inconveniently at
three in the afternoon to give my father a shower, she dismissed
them for good. Only one of my father's old colleagues managed
to penetrate her thicket of self-reliance: he called my father
directly and arranged to take him out to lunch every other week.

My mother's blood pressure rose. She was dizzy and nause-
ated during the day and couldn't eat. At night she couldn't sleep.

On the phone in California, I listened to her weeping—my
formidable, dominant mother, whom in fifty years I'd rarely seen
cry, and who so often heard me weep—as the long winter rains
fell outside my window. I felt tied to her misery like a dog tied to a
rattling can by a three-thousand-mile-long string. I, too, could not
sleep. In a *Physicians' Desk Reference* I bought at a garage sale, I
discovered that the entry for Ambien (the drug she was taking
for sleeplessness) listed dizziness, anxiety, and anorexia among its
side effects and "adverse events." I read the list aloud to her over
the phone, and to my relief she agreed to quit, and did.

I sent her a soothing book called *Sabbath,* which I hoped
would encourage her to rest, and a guided-imagery relaxation
tape. I fruitlessly nagged her to sign up for a yoga class and to
hire a caregiver. And every three or four months, whenever she
grew too thin, sleepless, or tearful, I flew east.

Thus I became part of the roll-aboard generation—the legions
of long-distance daughters and the smaller contingent of sons
who hoard their frequent-flier miles and often, but never often
enough, roll their suitcases on and off planes. The rest of the
time, we hire caregivers long-distance, do Internet research on
treatments and nursing homes, and try to make phone calls,
e-mail, and even Webcams substitute for being there. We make

up a substantial part of the nearly twenty-four million sons and daughters—about 8 percent of the U.S. population—who help care for aging parents.

I was grateful I could help my parents. I was amazed I wanted to. And I was scared.

One woman I knew spent twenty thousand dollars on airfare to Florida in a single year of dual parental medical crises. A man I knew insisted, after too many emergency flights east, that his father move into an excellent retirement home in our neighborhood called The Redwoods. The old man missed his friends and hated the food and the fog. Another woman quit her job to move in with her demented father and found herself impoverished and nearly homeless when the house was sold after his death to pay his debts. Some European countries pay family caregivers modestly and contribute to their pension funds to make up for what they lose by reducing their hours in the workforce. Not the United States.

A generation or two earlier, my path would have been clearly marked. I'd have moved into my parents' house, eaten the food at their table, and taken up the ancient burden of unpaid female altruism. It was a role women were once born for: the devoted wife, the selfless daughter-in-law, the uncomplaining, impoverished maiden aunt, and the unmarried daughter like Emily Dickinson, who stayed in her parents' home throughout their dying years and wrote her poems shuttered in an upstairs bedroom.

But even though our parents are more likely than ever to live long in fragile health, we baby-boom sons and daughters are often ill-equipped to help. Many of us no longer live close by or in extended families like my South African sheep-farming relatives, whose old folks would move to a smaller cottage when the son took over the farm and would help with grandchildren until they needed help themselves. Thanks partly to higher rates of divorce, 37 percent of baby-boom women are single; most rely on their own paychecks and many are poorly prepared for their own retirements. Married women aren't necessarily better off: few husbands still earn the breadwinner wages that in the 1950s and 1960s allowed many working-class and middle-class wives to stay home or work part-time while taking care of children, grandparents, parents, and parents-in-law. Men do more than they once did, but women still do most of the hands-on caregiving.

I was among the comparatively lucky ones. I had no children who needed me. I wasn't in debt. I owned a home and was covering its mortgage by renting it out while living with Brian. He was healthy, and his two sons were away at college and poised at the brink of adulthood. My work as a freelancer was flexible enough to let me drop everything for a week or two—without pay, that is. But I was time-stretched and money-stretched in ways that my mother and my grandmothers had not been.

I'd spent half my life in California, the land of backbreaking mortgages, benefit-free independent contractor gigs, expressive individualism, and personal reinvention, where the word "should" was a no-no and family obligations supposedly optional, like contracts written in water. No image of filial devotion from my storehouse of cultural clichés could guide me. Night after night, I was torn between the overpowering call of my blood and my life as a writer. When in California, I would worry about my parents and yearn to be with them; when in Middletown, I would worry about money and work, miss Brian, and want to go home. I didn't know which felt worse: abandoning my life or abandoning my parents. And so, for what turned out to be eight years, I would alternate between the two.

Before my father's stroke, I would answer the phone only when I felt like it. Afterward, I picked up no matter when it rang. When I woke before dawn with Brian snoring softly at my side and my brain wildly spinning solutions to my parents' problems, I would try to lull myself back to sleep by repeating the closest thing Buddhism has to a prayer, the Metta Sutta:

> May I be peaceful and at ease
> May I be filled with loving kindness
> May I be free from fear and danger
> May I be happy.

When that didn't work, I would sometimes try to remember the Twenty-Third Psalm or the Russian Orthodox "Jesus prayer" that I read long ago in *Franny and Zooey*, even though its theological underpinnings were alien to me:

> Lord Jesus Christ,
> Son of God
> Have mercy on me,
> A sinner.

I flew to Connecticut three times that first year—in early spring, midsummer, and fall—each time trying to make things a little better. On my first visit in March, I sat with my parents as I always had, at their breakfast table. My father fed himself slowly with a special spoon. A suction device anchored his plate to a rubbery blue place mat. My mother had pinned a stretchy black ribbon to a checked dinner napkin, which he looped with difficulty over his head, protecting his shirt from his dribbles while saving them both from the humiliating sight of a plastic disability bib. When the meal was over, he carefully folded his napkin up with grave attention, patting it into shape with the back of his only hand. His continence had returned—he no longer needed to wear Depends at night or a thick pad during the day. He had trouble finding words and finishing sentences. The father I knew had improvised, adapted, and overcome. Now the only phrase he said easily was, "I can't," and he said it often.

My parents seemed stuck together with glue on that first visit. My mother had long called impatience one of her "besetting sins," and she leaped to finish his sentences for him and did things for him before he could try them himself. When I watched her brushing his teeth after breakfast, even though he'd seemed handy enough with his spoon, I squirmed and said nothing. I dared not cross her.

I was a believer in experts and mutual-help groups. I found a free caregivers support group at Middlesex Hospital and took my mother there. Because Medicare funds mainly one-to-one interactions between patients and medical staff, the hospital was not reimbursed. Some of the most important and least glamorous help our family got took place like this, in odd-shaped, underpaid, and unpaid interstices within the health care system.

My mother sat uneasily with me in the crowded, windowless room in a circle of Middletown women caring for husbands debilitated by cancer, stroke, and other incurable but not promptly fatal illnesses. A nurse led the group. One wife, with short red hair and a measure of ease, said she got regular massages, paid a home health aide to give her a weekly afternoon off, and had a cell phone so that she could leave the house without worrying too much. When it was my mother's turn, she said she was overwhelmed. I slid in an oblique reference to her brushing my father's teeth. The woman with the cell phone raised her eyebrows and wondered if my mother wasn't overdoing it. "Simply listening to other women tell how they were coping with ailing husbands—some angry, some frustrated, and really venting—was an eye-opener," my mother would write to my father's three sisters. "I came away realizing that I was doing too much for Jeff—and not letting him struggle through himself." The next morning, she refused to brush my father's teeth and walked away after laying out his clothes. He brushed his teeth sulkily and, after what he told us was "a tremendous struggle," got himself dressed.

Over tea at the kitchen table a couple of days before my flight left, my mother and I talked idly, as if my father weren't there, about what I would do if she died first. Would I move my father to The Redwoods or try somehow to keep him in Middletown, perhaps with me or a hired caregiver? Worriedly he asked us, "What are you talking about?"

I was tongue-tied in matters of the heart. I sometimes felt like the little boy in Hans Christian Andersen's *Snow Queen*, whose heart turned to ice after it was pierced by a shard from a mirror that emphasized a critical and spiteful view of the world. I liked to go at things sideways, quoting the morning paper, or poetry, or a self-help book.

But my father could no longer understand long strings of sentences.

I caught my breath. I was about to make a vow more deep and true than the wedding vows I took in my thirties and in my forties disavowed.

"If Val dies," I said slowly, looking directly at him and calling my mother by her first name, "I will take care of you."

My mother never returned to the caregiver support group. She couldn't spare the time, she said. Half a century after coming to America, she remained a stranger in a strange land. She never understood why my two brothers and I liked baring our lives to people to whom we'd never before been introduced. I called my brother Jonathan and vented, but I didn't press him to go east, at least not as hard as we both would later wish. My friends on the West Coast made all the right noises of sympathy, but few had ever met my parents, and none could take my father to the movies and give my mother a break. I thought of going behind her proud back and asking more of my father's former colleagues to take my father out to lunch regularly, but I was afraid she would find out.

At night I worried about her agony and my father's stasis. In the daytime I worked the Rolodex I'd assembled in a decade of reporting on health and human behavior, beating a trail to a geriatric social worker in Middletown and a retired doctor in West Hartford who consulted with families facing medical catastrophes. I missed work deadlines and had trouble coming up with bright new story ideas for magazines. My income dropped in half.

My parents went to the social worker and didn't think much of him. The catastrophe doctor came to the house and suggested my father get involved in regular water aerobics: the longer he stayed physically independent, the doctor told my mother, the longer she could keep my father out of a nursing home. My mother nodded, signed the check for two hundred dollars, closed the door, and never took my father to the pool. She was too overwhelmed, it seemed, by the day-to-day. So I flew back to Middletown again, and that is how I found myself sitting on my meditation bench in the midsummer of 2002 with my parents still stuck together with glue, my father stripped of his wallet and watch, and my mother slapping at a fly with her flip-flop.

After breakfast, I drove my father to the Red Cross office downtown and filled out the application for the free paratransit van-ride service, cramming the lines with the list of his myriad disabilities. When we got home, I asked my mother for his Wesleyan ID and wallet—to my quiet surprise, she handed them over without resistance—and drove him to the Wesleyan pool, where I helped him show his ID to the attendant. Once inside, I swam laps while he strenuously pumped his knees up and down in the water at the shallow end, doing the physical therapy exercises he'd been taught in rehabilitation.

On Monday and Tuesday, I got the Red Cross van to pick us both up at home and take us to the pool. On Wednesday and Thursday, I put my father on the van by himself, drove to the pool to meet him, swam with him, put him back on the van, and met him back home. In his short-sleeved shirt, carrying his swimsuit in a drawstring bag, he looked like a little boy coming home from day camp, and I felt a wave of motherly, protective tenderness.

With the excuse that he needed to be on time for the van, I drove him to Pelton's Drugstore on Main Street and bought him a waterproof Timex with a black woven plastic band, to replace the stainless-steel one my mother had taken away. The next Monday, as I swam my laps and he did his water-walking, he looked over the string of floats and said, in a burst of eloquence—he often spoke better when my mother wasn't there— "You know, this is something I could really come to enjoy." He looked at his watch. "It's so nice having a watch."

That moment was more important to me than most of the articles I'd ever written, more valuable than the awards on my bookshelf and the hunk of Lucite engraved with my name. My self-confidence took a leap, and so did my capacity for unconditional love.

By the time I'd packed to leave one midsummer morning, my father was taking the van to the pool three mornings a week, doing his water aerobics on his own, and enlisting random strangers in the locker room to help him put on his shirt. One tiny, mundane, nontechnological intervention—water aerobics—had set a chain of good things in motion, helping him construct a life of small but real independent pleasures. It wasn't a life I'd have wanted to prolong unnaturally had it been mine, but it was his own.

The day my plane left, my mother's eyes filled with tears and she told me she didn't want me to go—a first. After years of competitive jousting, we'd finally worked together as a team. "If only you lived closer," she said, stroking my hand at the kitchen table. "If only you lived an hour and a half away. If only you lived in Boston."

I'd wanted to hear her speak like this—the softness, the need, the appreciation—for much of my life. For a moment I wished I could stay.

For fifty years I'd watched her take on tasks that overwhelmed me. Nothing stopped her—not leaving everyone she'd known and loved in South Africa, in a doomed society where African servants brought tea trays to the bedroom door each morning; not raising three children in postwar Britain with a one-armed husband who couldn't change a diaper; not arriving almost friendless on the docks of New York in 1957 with a couple of trunks and one good blue wool Jaeger suit.

In the midcentury modern house she and my father built overlooking a lake in the suburbs of Boston, she'd painted the front door turquoise and in the long window beside it hung strings of orange-juice-can lids strung from nylon fishing lines. The disks caught the light like glittering golden scales: a work of art, ingenious, and practically free. She stepped back for a look, arms akimbo, with a paint smudge on one cheek and a blond tendril falling from her French twist, and sang her favorite line from *Annie Get Your Gun*: "Anything you can do, I can do better! I can do anything better than you!"

Decades later, I still felt like a clumsy teenager in her presence. And now that teenager was supposed to become her parents' parent. I stroked my mother's hand, told her that families were never meant to live this far apart, and went upstairs to get my bag.

*   *   *

In California a few weeks later, I got a letter of thanks from a man who, much to my surprise, could think, read, and write even though he could barely speak.

"Not only did you do what you said you were going to do, but you did it with great panache, which the French claim they have lots of," said my father in a letter he'd probably labored over for hours on his computer, his written eloquence utterly and amazingly at odds with the smiling, inarticulate man I kissed good-bye at the airport near Hartford. Although the stroke had blasted his capacity for understanding and articulating spoken language, it apparently spared places in his brain, highly developed thanks to decades of academic work, where neurons process visual data and are at least partly responsible for the ability to read and write.

"One of those ways was your ingenious devices for achieving things like the organizing of the swimming," his letter went on. "The drivers were touched by your familiarity. You were never at a loss for a plan when something went wrong. There was a sadness in your leaving which could not be avoided. You made your Mother and me very sad, but also very proud. We left the airport in a strange but wonderful mood. So you did what you had to do without causing any fuss. So my darling, that is what I want to say. All my love to you. If I have been guilty in the past of being ungrateful, then I must try to make it good."

Below the printed text, in a tangle of spidery lines, barely decipherable, my father had written his first name.

CHAPTER 3

RITES OF PASSAGE

In the fall of 2002, my father quietly turned eighty with no particular celebration beyond a handwritten note from my mother and a letter from me. With the doggedness that is part of his legacy to me, he'd settled for little victories and accepted losses. In the year since the stroke, he learned again how to fasten his belt and to comb his own hair, despite his now-limited reach, using a special long-handled comb I ordered from a disability catalog against my mother's wishes; she hated the way it screamed "handicap." Three times a week he walked to the pool to do his water exercises, slightly dragging one foot—my mother had canceled the Red Cross van because it sometimes brought him home late after leaving off other passengers in a neighboring town. Twice a month, his former colleague Richard Adelstein took him to lunch, doing most of the talking while my father did most of the listening. With encouragement from Angela, his speech therapist, he set to work on an autobiography. But the gains were slowing, as the rehabilitation center brochure had said they would. He was settling in at a new baseline—with the memories, mind, and reading comprehension of a highly educated eighty-year-old; the spoken speech of a four- or five-year-old; and the physical dependence of a six-year-old.

I spent Thanksgiving of 2002 in western Massachusetts with Brian, his sister Ann and her family, and Brian's eighty-eight-year-old father John. John had advanced arthritis and had suffered a minor stroke; because he now needed a walker to get around the house and a stair glide to go up stairs, he'd vacated his house in Queens and moved in with his daughter's family. (Four months later we would fly east for his funeral.) After spending a week caring for him while Ann and her husband took a vacation, Brian and I drove to Middletown, where I introduced him to my parents for the first time.

I was afraid they'd think he wasn't good enough for me, and to tell the truth, I had my doubts. He wore 49ers sweatshirts and baseball caps, made his living as a medical salesman, and sometimes said things like "it's raining cats and buckets" or "the candidate didn't pass the mustard." His first forays into connecting with my parents hadn't gone well. When he told my mother over the phone how wonderful her daughter was, she'd said, "Well, she's a handful." When, at a family lunch in a restaurant, he asked my father for permission to marry me, my father had grinned, shaken his head, and said—and I will never know to the end of my days whether he was toying with Brian or saying an uncomfortable, stroke-freed truth—"You're just not suitable!"

I needn't have worried. My father took Brian on a tour of the Wesleyan campus, just the two of them, and in the end neither he nor my mother could resist Brian's persistent goodwill. Only after their deaths would I learn, from reading the enthusiastic

letters that my mother wrote to relatives in South Africa, just
how happy they were made by how happy Brian made me.

After Brian left, my father and I walked down one morning
to the Wesleyan pool. The lifeguards had come to expect him,
and they set out the disability hoist to lift him, like a lineman in
a bucket, in and out of the water. On the way home to the house
on Pine Street, he told me he was "on permanent holiday." Long
before his stroke, he'd become expert in enduring what he could
not change—from his lost arm to his sons' emotional distance
to my mother's chronic discontent—and he used that capacity
now.

Meanwhile, my mother had grown. A retired Wesleyan math
professor taught her how to balance her checkbook, and once a
month she took it down to her tax accountant's office, where a
bookkeeper helped her chase down the errors that set her totals
off by a dollar or two. A neighbor, a former social worker, suggested she make a list of the caregiving tasks she abhorred, and
hire someone. Through the Wesleyan grapevine, she found a
dignified older African-American woman named Annie, and for
ten dollars a visit, Annie came in and gave my father a shower
three mornings a week.

But just as things stabilized, my parents' lawyer, an old family
friend, advised my mother to sell the house and buy into a "life
care community" before my father got too addled or helpless to
qualify. My father was not going to get better, she said. He was
going to get worse. Panicked and sleepless, my mother towed my
father around assisted living places, rejecting one for its Jell-O and
Lutheran religiosity, others for their distance from any towns, and
still others for their predominance of Republicans in golf pants.

She was still on the banks of vigorous, early old age, on the
far side of the river from my father's helpless desolation. She
didn't want to trade her autonomous though burdened life—her
friends, her garden, her sewing room, her weekly trips to Freddy's

Middlesex Fruitery on Main Street for the crispest green apples and freshest red oak lettuce—for an expensive, overheated shoe box of an apartment, with overcooked food, in what she called a "henhouse." But she was terrified of running out of money and of disasters she couldn't foresee, and exhausted by maintaining the house and its acre of trees and grounds while taking care of my father. To my dismay, she'd already had a real estate agent in to price the house. Our family had lost so much; I did not want to lose that house as well—that island of beauty and order, that reminder of the life my brothers and I had once lived.

Armed with a referral from the catastrophe doctor, I drove my parents to West Hartford to meet a new lawyer, this one a pioneer in a specialty called "elder law." He was a ferrety little man in his forties with a straw mustache. His own father had been struck by Alzheimer's disease in his late fifties. By the time the old man died in a nursing home, there was nothing left for his widow or children.

The lawyer sat us down at a blond conference table and told my parents to transfer all the mutual funds they held outside their IRAs into my name. If my father had to enter a nursing home, we would first "spend down" their IRAs. Then Medicaid, the program intended for the poor, would pick up his bills, just as it covers 45 percent of the more than $137 billion that the nation spends annually on long-term care. If my parents didn't sequester some money, the lawyer said, my mother would risk what he called "spousal impoverishment." Medicaid would not cover my father's nursing care until they spent down most of their assets.

If, on the other hand, some money was moved promptly into my name, that money could be used to pay for my mother's care when she got frail, and perhaps even for an inheritance for my brothers and me. The scheme, I hoped, would give my mother a backup plan and stop her stampede toward assisted living. She could stay in the house that felt like an anchor to us, hire more help, and manage on her own.

"Do it now," the lawyer said, fingering his mustache. Changes in the law were afoot to make what we were contemplating more difficult. Technically, the scheme was not illegal: parents transfer assets to adult children legitimately all the time, and as long as my father needed no Medicaid help for at least three years (since extended to five) nobody would scrutinize the financial transfer.

It was the sort of thing my father, when he could speak, would have called "sharp practice." He sat in a chair, a compliant, voiceless witness.

The lawyer laid out a sheaf of documents for us to sign, far more extensive (and expensive) than the living wills and "durable power of attorney for health care" documents they'd signed years earlier. First came updated wills and new "advanced directives" declaring that they wanted no life-sustaining treatment if they were in comas or likely to die within six months. (The documents said nothing, I'd later realize, about dementia or tiny internalized life-support devices like pacemakers.) Then came new "durable power of attorney for health care" forms, giving my mother and me the authority to make my father's medical decisions when, in the sole opinion of the family doctor, he could no longer make his own. Finally, there were documents entrusting me with my mother's medical guardianship, power-of-attorney forms giving my mother and me free rein over my father's financial affairs, and similar ones giving me comparable authority regarding my mother.

My mother showed my father where to sign, and in his new, oddly miniaturized and rickety hand, he did. He'd been the family money manager and the ballast to my mother's volatile, wind-filled sails—her rock and our paterfamilias. Now, with my brothers still keeping their distance in California, shards of his shattered role were falling to her and to me, his disorganized, bright, well-meaning daughter.

As the notary turned the long legal pages and busied herself with her stamps, I looked at the language that foreshadowed our new world. We had no idea just how flimsy these paper amulets would turn out to be.

After my mother and I called Fidelity and set the money transfer in motion, I took my father for a walk in the forest surrounding Colonel Clarence Wadsworth's turn-of-the-twentieth-century wedding-cake mansion recently refurbished by the city of Middletown. My parents and I had walked its woods and streams for decades, flouting the nuns in the days when it was a private religious retreat center run by Our Lady of the Cenacle. I held his hand. He dragged his right foot. Autumn leaves lay everywhere.

I asked him if his life was still worth living.

"Are you talking about *Do Not Resuscitate*?" he asked pronouncing it *Re-Sus-Ki-Tate*. I wasn't thinking that specifically, but I nodded anyway.

He said my mother would have been better off if he'd died of his stroke. "She'd have weeped the weep of a widow," he said in his garbled, poststroke speech. "And then she would have been all right."

As we shuffled through the fallen leaves, I thought of my paternal grandmother Alice, whom I'd hardly known. She died in 1963, at the age of eighty-three, on the custodial wing of a South African hospital, the first of our family to die among strangers. Five years of devastating strokes had left her so incontinent, incoherent, and angry that she refused to eat, and her devoted husband, Ernest, and his unmarried sister Mary had been forced to stop caring for her at home.

Alice's years of lingering misery—then a far rarer pathway to death than it is today—provoked a spiritual crisis in several of my father's four siblings, and they openly wondered why God was punishing her this way. "The noises she made were impossible to interpret . . . and did little for my always wavering faith in a merciful God," my late uncle Guy, a well-known South African poet, wrote in his memoir about her last, worst years. Within hours of her death, he stood with my stunned grandfather at the foot of her bed, contemplating her fixed sightless eyes and emptied form. "She was no longer the painful parody of what she once had been," Guy wrote. "She was dead, blessedly dead, and free at last, beyond the agony of fumbling for words and meanings in an eighty-three-year-old body."

Her husband, my grandfather Ernest, died in 1965 at the age of seventy-nine, at the tail end of times when medicine did not routinely stave off death among the very old. He went to his backyard wood shop one day, completed a set of chairs he'd left unfinished for thirty years, cleaned off his workbenches, had a heart attack, and died two days later in a plain hospital bed.

Holding my father's soft, mottled hand, I vainly wished him a similar merciful death.

"Losing my—arm. W-w-w-ugh. W-w-ugh. W-w-w-w-ugh. One thing," my father said, gesturing, trapped in the prison of his damaged speech. I understood: after a day or two in the army field hospital in a state of suicidal despair, and after months of rehabilitation and countless nights drinking on the Rhodes University campus with other wounded and demobilized veterans, he'd picked himself up, abandoned his hoped-for career in chemistry, reeducated himself as a historian, met and married my mother, and made a good life.

"R-r-r-ugh. R-r-r-ugh. Rotator—." He shrugged, and again I understood. In his sixties, a tear in his rotator cuff, repaired surgically without much benefit, had left him unable to reach the salt across the table. But he'd adapted. He'd still been my dear father Jeff.

"But *this*," he said, looking me straight in the eye and shaking his head in puzzlement and outrage. *This* was different.

"*This.*"

Back at the house, I hung up his coat by the door. The hook was too high for his now-limited reach, and my mother didn't want to move it down and spoil the clean lines of the vestibule. Upstairs in the cold guest bedroom, I sat down at her old calligraphy desk, pulling a blanket over my knees. My mind was still moving in conflicted ways: I hoped my father would die a natural death; I wanted him to be as functional and happy as possible. Running my finger down the numbers in the "physical therapy" section of the Greater Hartford Yellow Pages, I found a physical therapist in nearby Cromwell with her own exercise pool who accepted Medicare's low reimbursement rates. I wrote the number on an index card, handed it to my mother triumphantly, and started packing my Rollaboard for California, thus setting in motion a fix with devastating, unforeseen consequences.

II

FAST MEDICINE

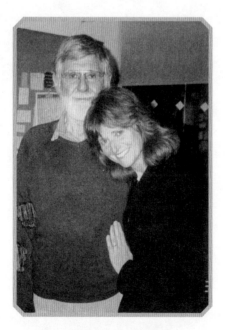

Jeffrey and Katy Butler

CHAPTER 4

THE TYRANNY OF HOPE

In early December, my mother called with news. The enthusiastic new physical therapist had sent my father through his pool exercises so hard that two gaps had opened up in the smooth muscle of his lower abdomen. Through those gaps nosed bits of fat and tissue, making painful humps beneath the skin. The humps—technically known as inguinal hernias—were easily fixable with the latest laparoscopic surgery, to be performed under general anesthesia. Dr. Fales recommended a truss to temporarily ease the pain, but my mother balked because its $200 cost was not covered by Medicare. Time was of the essence: without a surgical fix or at least a truss, a loop of small intestine might get pinched or "incarcerated" in the wall of my father's abdomen, lose its blood supply, and develop gangrene. In my ignorance, I figured that a hernia repair was too minor to warrant my dropping work and making a trip east. Only later would I understand that there is no such thing as minor surgery for the very old and frail.

Dr. Fales referred my father to a local general surgeon, who sent him to a cardiologist for a preoperative clearance. On the day after Christmas, a little more than a year after the stroke, my mother drove my father down to the Connecticut shore for an urgent appointment with Dr. John Rogan of Middlesex Cardiology Associates. Dr. Rogan was fifty-two, a mild-mannered man with dark hair and a receding hairline, a graduate of the University of Massachusetts Medical School, and a Catholic. His clinical notes would describe my father as "a pleasant South African gentleman" who "fought for the British in WWII and lost his left arm to a mortar blast in the Italian campaign." Years later he would write me a letter describing how much he'd liked him.

Dr. Rogan saw nothing unusual in my father's clinical case. He ran an electrocardiogram and discovered that at rest, my father's aging heart beat only thirty-five times a minute—a little more than half the rate of most healthy young people. Technically known as "asymptomatic bradycardia," my dad had had the condition for at least six years. It is common among the very athletic and the very old. Many Olympic endurance athletes have slow resting heart rates because their large, efficient hearts pump large volumes of oxygen-saturated blood to their muscles during contests and then slow down radically when at rest.

My father's heart was slow because he was eighty.

His heart's natural pacemaker, a comma-shaped bundle of nerve fibers called the sinoatrial node, had, in the process of normal aging, lost much of its firing power. Perched near the top of the upper-right chamber of the heart, the sinoatrial node is about the size of a pencil eraser. Day and night, from birth to death, it spontaneously fires a tiny electrical charge, pauses, gathers itself, and fires again. The signal pulses down through heart muscle and nerve fibers to the ventricles, the twin major lower pumping chambers, cueing them to squeeze blood out into the arteries for transport to all the limbs and vital organs. By the age of seventy-five, the sinoatrial node has often lost as much as 90 percent of its cells through a natural process of aging and cell die-off. Nerve cells elsewhere in the heart's electrical conduction system have thinned out as well.

My father's slow heartbeat first revealed itself in 1994, during a routine electrocardiogram at his internist's office. Sometimes the signals pulsing from his sinoatrial node took a few extra seconds to reach the lower chambers. Sometimes his heart paused between beats. Once in a while it missed beats altogether, a pattern cardiologists call a Wenckebach rhythm. But despite the wrong sort of squiggle on the electrocardiogram—a pattern that Dr. Rogan would call "first degree heart block" and "Sick Sinus Syndrome"—my dad had never fainted or gotten dizzy or showed any other sign of heart trouble, aside from an occasional puffy ankle. If he'd grown old before the pacemaker was invented, nobody would have called his heart diseased—just worn out.

Dr. Rogan looked at the tests and decided that my father needed a pacemaker. Without a "pacer," he said, my father's heart might stop under the stress of general anesthesia during the hernia surgery. A sense of urgency, combined with the assumption that the treatment offered has no alternatives and no downsides, are common ingredients in medical decisions, later regretted, involving the fragile elderly. It was the second time that Dr. Rogan had seen my father, and the second time he'd recommended a pacemaker.

Dr. Rogan had first examined my father a year earlier, in November of 2001, just weeks before the first stroke, after my father's gastroenterologist became alarmed by my Dad's slow heartbeat.

Dr. Rogan had told my dad then that he "did qualify for a pace-maker," even though cardiology treatment guidelines did not actually recommend one for asymptomatic bradycardia. In a later letter to me, Dr. Rogan would call my father's case then "a gray zone to be sure, and not fitting neatly into the guidelines. I felt he should consider a pacer before any major symptom, thinking it inevitable he would need one."

My then-vigorous and intact father told Dr. Rogan that he wasn't interested unless a pacemaker was absolutely necessary— and nor was his internist, Dr. Fales, who considered it overtreat-ment. Dr. Rogan made plans nevertheless to hook my father up to a portable Holter cardiac monitor, a strap-on electrocardio-graph that can record the heart rhythm twenty-four hours a day. The longer test period might have uncovered further rhythmic oddities and strengthened the case for a device. But before the Holter test could take place, my mother had called Dr. Rogan's office in tears to say my father had had his first stroke.

At about the same time that Dr. Rogan first broached the idea of a pacemaker for my dad, a cardiologist in Italy named Alberto Dolara was promoting a new clinical approach he called "Slow Medicine." Fast medicine, like fast food, he wrote in an internationally influential essay published in a leading Italian cardiology journal in early 2002, often involved a barrage of rap-idly prescribed tests and treatments—fixing rather than heal-ing. Slow medicine, like slow food, valued restraint, calm, and above all, time: time to weigh the emotional and physical costs of medical treatment; time to evaluate new methods and tech-nologies; time, as the end of life approached, to stop frenetic *doing* and to take care instead of the broader needs of patients and their families.

Excessive eagerness to act, Dolara wrote later in English in

Acta Cardiologica, can result in "premature timing in surgery, too much enthusiasm for new technologies, exaggerated emphasis on tests . . . and scarce attention to the needs of patients." "To do more," wrote one of his Slow Medicine colleagues, Francesco Fiorista, elsewhere, "is not necessarily to do better."

The Italian doctors were part of a quietly emerging medical counterculture drawing mainly from such money-starved and unglamorous domains as geriatrics, palliative care, internal and family medicine, and hospice care. If the movement had a birth date, it was probably 1967, when an English nurse named Cicely Saunders opened the first modern hospice, St. Christopher's, in London, with the goal of treating a patient's "total suffering" rather than trying to extend life. In many ways, Slow Medicine represented not an advance, but a return to ancient ways of doctoring

Even though the Slow Medicine movement—which broadly speaking emphasizes patient-centered care, unrushed medical decisions and "care" over "cure"—was quietly mushrooming, its philosophy was easy to ignore amid the clangor of better-funded, high-tech medicine, with its dramatic fixes and sometimes exaggerated hopes. The Italian doctors were in the minority— especially among cardiologists—but they were not outliers, and nor was my medically cautious father. Some studies suggest that patients are more likely than their doctors to reject major elective surgery when fully informed of pros, cons, and alternatives—information that nearly half of patients say they don't get. And although Dr. Rogan assumed it was an unbridled good thing to extend my father's life, nearly a third of the severely ill and dependent don't feel that way. In a 1997 study in *The Journal of the American Geriatrics Society,* 30 percent of seriously ill people surveyed in a hospital said they would "rather die" than live permanently in nursing homes—a preference that neither their doctors nor their close relatives were much good at predicting. In another study, 28 percent of people with congestive heart failure said they'd trade a single day of life in excellent health for two years of survival in their current condition.

When my parents met with Dr. Rogan in late 2002, with my father now stroke-damaged and in pain from his hernias, they had unwittingly arrived at an unmarked crossroads where even the most seemingly routine medical decisions become fraught and sacred. Assumptions that went unquestioned when my dad was whole and vigorous—when "saving his life" meant more than exchanging one pathway to death for another—were starting to shift. The decision that day was not simply *how* or *when* to treat, but *whether*. My parents were contemplating more than a pacemaker. They were contemplating how much suffering they would bear in exchange for more time together on earth. And they did not know it.

At this crossroads, each miraculous life-extending technology pulls up from the depths a tangle of our most deeply held and unarticulated moral questions and puts them under a halogen light. How grateful are we for the gift of life and what are we willing to undergo for more of it? Would we rather die too soon or too late? How do we make sense of the loss of human bonds that death brings even to those who believe in heaven? Does a caregiver's suffering have moral standing? Can a daughter express her love for her father by doing all she can to let him die, or is that an expression of her selfishness and buried hate?

What would my father have said that day at Dr. Rogan's office if the pacemaker had been discussed as a choice-point rather than as a necessity? What if Dr. Rogan had told him that its battery would last ten years? What would my mother have said if the doctor had asked her how she was coping with caregiving? What if Dr. Rogan had asked my father whether he felt his life was still worth living?

I do not know. Dr. Rogan was a specialist in heart rhythm, not in geriatrics, psychiatry, or family medicine. He clearly cared about his patients, and his approach to my father's case conformed to accepted medical practice. He was simply tightly focused on one fixable piece of my father's problems. If he hadn't suggested the pacemaker and something had gone wrong, our family could even have sued him for negligence for failing to meet the "standard of care" in our local community. And how was he to know? He was presented with a wife—my mother—who knew how to keep up appearances. My father could not easily follow an animated dinner-table conversation then, much less talk with a near-stranger about how he wanted to die, or live. And in my parents' eyes, I was just a daughter with problems of her own on a faraway coast—struggling to earn a living, growing warily closer to a new man, and negotiating a sometimes fraught relationship with his two nearly grown sons, who were accustomed to having the run of their father's house.

My mother was not a compliant or stupid woman. She wasn't enthusiastic about the pacemaker and she knew that their internist, the trusted Dr. Fales, opposed it. But she was anxious to get my father out of pain and was no expert on high-tech medicine. In the course of her long life, she usually believed what doctors told her, and on the whole it had worked out well. She grew up in times when almost all doctors practiced what the Italians had taken to calling Slow Medicine: they made house calls, earned incomes roughly equal to those of their patients, served the same families for decades, didn't get gifts from drug and device salesmen, and didn't prescribe technologies they indirectly profited from. She was in her thirties in the 1950s when my brothers and I were inoculated with Jonas Salk's polio vaccine, developed for the benefit of all humankind and never patented, saving lives by the millions. She knew medicine had changed since then. She once said to me, "The whole fifteen-minute game—it's a joke, sweetheart, it's not medicine!" But she wasn't the type to come to an appointment with an Internet printout.

And so the system rewarded nobody for saying "no" or even "wait"—not even my frugal, intelligent, *Consumer Reports*–reading mother. Medicare and supplemental insurance covered almost every penny of my father's pacemaker even though they would not cover a cent of a temporary truss that might have bought us time for an informed decision. My mother asked more questions and was given more government-mandated consumer information when she bought a new Camry a year later.

There was more. There is a school of thought that maintains that if patients educate themselves and sign all the right forms, they'll escape the unhappy medical outcomes they dread. But my mother was not just a medical consumer. She was an agonized, exhausted, and still-hopeful wife. She had told my father that he was *not* to die first and leave her alone. She saw his stroke as a setback to overcome, not as the first loosening of a mooring on a boat that would sail out to sea without her and sink. "I was not ready for his dying then," she would tell me much later, when she came to regret her decision that day. "I still had hope we could improve things. I hadn't really taken in that once you've had one stroke, you're likely to have another."

Dr. Fales watched from the sidelines. He knew there were things worse than dying. His own father had recently been diagnosed with Alzheimer's disease. "If it had been my dad, I'd have talked to my mom and said, 'It's time,'" he would tell me later, after both my parents were dead. "'The pacemaker is going to extend his life into a period when he has no reason to live. Enough is enough. Let nature take its course.'"

But my mother did not call Dr. Fales.

She shrugged and said yes. The pacemaker surgery was scheduled for the following week, and she called to let me know. I bit my lip. It is one thing to silently wish that your father's heart might fail. It's another to actively abet his death by opposing surgery.

The effects of these decisions rippled through our lives for the next six years.

Dr. Fales, who loved my parents and understood their suffering far better than Dr. Rogan did, was notified by fax. As he remembers it, he gave Dr. Rogan a call—a call Dr. Rogan doesn't remember getting. "Because the surgeon and the cardiologist went a couple of extra years in their training, my opinion didn't weigh in heavily, even though I knew Jeff better than anyone else," he told me later. He worried, too, that if surgery was further delayed, my father's hernias might become gangrenous. "That would have been dire," he said. "They put Jeff in a bind, and I gave up."

And had Dr. Fales not given up? Medicare would have effectively penalized him. It would have paid Dr. Fales nothing for phone calls to the specialists, just fifty-four dollars for a fifteen-minute office visit with my parents, and only an extra twenty to forty dollars if he sent in paperwork justifying a longer meeting. A payment of two hundred dollars for such talks was proposed as part of health care reform in 2009, but after distortion by a consultant for the conservative Hudson Institute think tank, it was widely decried as reimbursement for "death panels" and stripped from the bill. As a result, doctors of all sorts, especially oncologists, are reimbursed well for administering close-to-futile second- and third-line treatments and reimbursed hardly at all—financially punished, in fact—if they take the time to explain the case for doing less.

Both Dr. Rogan and Dr. Fales believed that without a pacemaker, my father would probably not have lived for more than another two years. His aging heart, Dr. Fales later told me, would probably have gradually become slower and more arrhythmic. If he were lucky, it would have paused too long one night and never started again. If he were unlucky, he'd have had fainting spells and fallen and broken a hip or even cracked his skull.

One way or another, his brain, kidneys, and other vital organs would have slowly failed, starved of sufficient oxygen.

"Finally the heart would have just stopped beating," Dr. Fales said. "He would have died peacefully. But nowadays we don't get to see this natural course much, because everybody gets devices." Not having a pacemaker would not have guaranteed my father a quick or easy death. But having a pacemaker deprived him of his best chance for one.

On the afternoon of January 2, 2003, my father was wheeled into an operating room at Middlesex Memorial Community Hospital in Middletown. His chest was numbed with a local anesthetic. Dr. Jonathan Aranow, a popular local surgeon specializing in laparoscopic surgery who trained at Harvard Medical School and Beth Israel Deaconess hospital in Boston, made a three-inch cut in the diagonal groove below my father's right collarbone and opened his cephalic vein, which runs near the surface of the skin in the upper arm and leads to the heart. Guided by the image from a fluoroscope—a sort of real-time motion-picture X-ray—Dr. Aranow threaded a long, spiraling wire, called a lead, down the vein and into the apex of the right ventricle, the lower pumping chamber of my father's heart. Next Dr. Aranow inserted a second lead down the same vein into my father's right atrium, the smaller upper chamber. Once both leads were in place, the surgeon fastened the ends of the wires to the plastic top of the pacemaker's flat, metallic pulse generator, which looked a bit like a Zippo lighter. Two weeks later, he fixed my father's hernias under general anesthetic.

Medicare paid Dr. Aranow $461 for the forty-five-minute pacemaker operation, and the hospital a lump sum of about $12,000, of which the lion's share, about $7,500, went to St. Jude Medical of St. Paul, Minnesota, the world's second-largest manufacturer of pacemakers, defibrillators, and other cardiac-rhythm devices. St. Jude is a major player in Minnesota's "Medical Alley," a thriving cluster of medical technology companies that includes the behemoth Medtronic.

I cannot tell you precisely what the hospital paid St. Jude for the pacemaker, nor could Dr. Rogan or Dr. Aranow. The hospital told me only that St. Jude was its standard brand, as Middlesex is part of a regional consortium of hospitals that negotiates purchases in bulk. The makers of cardiac devices require hospitals to sign agreements that keep negotiated prices secret even from the doctors who prescribe the devices. Thus buffered from open competition and the law of supply and demand, pacemaker prices—85 percent of them picked up indirectly by Medicare—have declined only slightly over the past half century, in contrast, for instance, to the prices of digital cameras. Prices vary widely: according to a U.S. Government Accountability Office study published in 2012, one hospital paid $8,723 more than another for the same complex cardiac-rhythm device.

With threads of fine strong silk, Dr. Aranow sewed the pacemaker into a pocket of skin below my father's collarbone. Hidden from sight were its electronic innards: a tiny lithium battery, the electric pulse generator, and a miniscule computer capable of sensing any variation in my father's heart rhythm. The first wire resting in my father's atrium sensed his every atrial heartbeat. The second wire delivered a tiny jolt of electric current to his ventricle whenever the natural beat slowed, keeping the heart muscle squeezing and synchronized at a steady seventy-five beats per minute. The little gizmo, one of millions now pulsing in hearts around the world, began sending out its signals a hundred thousand times each day and night. It was a thousand times lighter, safer, smaller, and smarter than the first device to continuously pace a human heart, more than sixty years ago.

CHAPTER 5

INVENTING LIFESAVING AND TRANSFORMING DEATH

The year was 1952; the place, Beth Israel Hospital in Boston. The internist and researcher Paul Zoll had spent the previous two years in the hospital's lab, experimenting with electrical shocks to stop and start the hearts of dogs. Now he wanted to try out what he'd learned on a human being. His first patient-subject was a man who'd been brought to the hospital emergency room on the brink of death, with the lower chambers of his heart quivering chaotically. Dr. Zoll applied his experimental shocking device to the man's chest in an attempt to stabilize his heart rhythm, but the patient was already bleeding fatally from a coronary vein punctured accidentally in a desperate attempt to inject adrenaline directly into his heart. He died in about twenty minutes.

Zoll's second patient, known to medical history only as "R.A.," was a sixty-five-year-old man with a history of cardiac disease whose heart was alternating between periods of standstill and flurries of rapid, irregular beats. Zoll came to R.A.'s bedside with a rolling cart holding a bulky off-the-shelf lab appliance, about the size and shape of a large metal bread box. Called a Grass Physiological Stimulator, the machine featured a front surface with rows of switches and dials and a coiled, heavily insulated cord that split in two before ending in a pair of electrified needles. Traditionally used in the hospital laboratory to study how nerve and muscle tissues responded to electrical stimulus, it was capable of delivering rhythmic, calibrated electric shocks.

Zoll plugged the Stimulator into a wall socket, stuck the two needle electrodes into the skin of R.A.'s chest, and delivered 130 volts of current. R.A.'s chest muscles convulsed, and the pulsing currents rippled through the chest wall to his heart. As long as the shocks continued, R.A.'s heart beat rhythmically, but whenever Zoll tried to dial down the charge, the heart stopped. For six days, the Stimulator paced R.A.'s heart as he ate, carried on conversations, and followed the World Series on the radio from his hospital bed. Finally his heart resumed beating on its own, at a slow but steady forty-four beats a minute. Zoll removed the electrodes, and some days later R.A. went home. He died ten months later outside the hospital after his diseased heart entered another flurry of disturbed rhythms.

Zoll wrote up R.A.'s case for the *New England Journal of Medicine*. The Stimulator was not a permanent solution. But for the first time ever, an electrical device had successfully managed the beating of a human heart without requiring a surgeon to cut deep into the chest wall.

Over the next three years, devices like the Stimulator, made by a company called Electrodyne, brought more of Zoll's desperate patients back from the brink. But many were not as lucky as R.A. The Stimulator was an emergency device—a crude, clunky, hospital-based "bridge" technology intended to carry a patient over a brief crisis. For those whose hearts never resumed normal rhythms, it offered a poor substitute for living. Tethered to electrical sockets and lying in hospital beds, these experimental Lazaruses sometimes grimaced as they suffered the Stimulator's intense repeated shocks and the powerful, involuntary chest contractions the shocks provoked. Sometimes the device burned and blistered the skin. Children subjected to it cried and screamed through heavy sedation.

In 1955 or 1956, about three years after R.A.'s miraculous revival, a group of interns and residents at Beth Israel visited the room of a chronic heart patient who "had been on an external Zoll pacemaker for a long period of time," in the words of the late Seymour Furman, then an intern and later a leading cardiac surgeon. "After a pep talk which the house staff, myself included, had given the patient about the wonders of the future to come, which we didn't believe and he equally didn't believe," Furman said later, the house staff left the room and the man "committed suicide by turning off the switch." It was the first known case of a patient refusing to submit to a life-extending cardiac machine—not a suicide exactly, but a relatively new moral act, one without its own name.

Such stories rarely reached the popular press, however, and they weren't the dominant notes. The mood of postwar America—including that of my own newly arrived, immigrant family—was optimistic, self-confident, iconoclastic, and fascinated with science. Faith in rationality, progress, and unbridled human experiment rivaled that of the Renaissance and the Enlightenment. When my family disembarked from the *Queen Elizabeth* on the docks of New York in 1957 and searched for the trunks holding my teddy bear and my father's typewriter, Dwight Eisenhower, a Second World War military hero, was president. The economy was booming. After seven years of austerity in England, we Butlers were making a fresh start in a brash young nation, set to build on the technological advances catalyzed by the Second World War.

My father found a job teaching in the African Studies program at Boston University. We rented a house in the suburbs with central heating, our first television, and a large unfenced yard. Our family stopped going to church. We bought a secondhand Buick that drove like a sofa, which my mother guided nervously down the new American superhighways, funded by an expanding federal government, to a supermarket where, to her amazement, she could buy oranges, dish soap, and frozen chicken under one enormous, brightly lit roof. After three years of renting, my parents bought land on the edge of a lake and decided to build a radically modern house with huge glass windows, a house a bit more expensive than they could afford.

Bulldozers brought in fill, and a concrete mixer poured its gray sludge into the foundation forms. The walls and windows came in pieces on a truck—giant panels of redwood and glass, erected in days like a house of cards. It was basically a box with a peaked roof, ample light, lots of sliding glass, a single bathtub, and four small upstairs bedrooms nestled under the eaves, but to us it was grand. Inspired in part by Frank Lloyd Wright's moderately priced Usonian House, our new home, called a Techbuilt, was an attempt to bring Bauhaus design to the masses. Costs were kept down with modular construction, an open plan in the downstairs living spaces, and a dearth of fine lines and carpenter's trim. The neighbors, in their reproduction Colonials, were shocked.

To save money, my parents acted as their own general contractors, hiring electricians and plumbers and doing much of the rest of the work themselves. On weekends and in the evenings, my father, who was also teaching full-time in Boston and racing to rewrite his PhD thesis, joined my mother in hanging Sheetrock, mudding joints, and painting walls. When it came time to tile the bathroom, my mother went off alone to a half-built housing development, watched the professional tilers at work, and came home and did the same things herself. I thought there was nothing she couldn't do.

My new bedroom window looked over the lake, and my brothers and I spent the summer there, sailing a secondhand Sailfish with a boldly striped, lateen-rigged sail woven out of Dacron, another radical modern innovation. We had little money for furniture, but my mother splurged, at a store called Design Research in Cambridge, on a Japanese lamp designed by Noguchi, a zigzagging column of paper and light, which she hung in a corner of the bare cork-floored living room, near two butterfly chairs, a cheap, foam-filled black couch, and a mosaic coffee table that she and my father built from a kit from the Door Store. Even her coffeemaker was modern and scientific: an hourglass-shaped beaker called a Chemex that looked like something from a chemistry lab.

John Kennedy was elected president. The *Jetsons* cartoon show premiered on television. NASA vowed to put a man on the moon, and Congress ordered the National Institutes of Health to fund the development of an entirely artificial heart.

All over the United States and in Europe, buoyed by the same postwar spirit, doctors and inventors working in garages and sheet-metal shops and hospital labs were cobbling together new medical contraptions and surgical devices from washing machines, vacuum cleaners, cattle watering tubs, glass tubing, orange-juice cans, and sausage casings. Materials invented or pressed into military service during the Second World War—nylon, Dacron, silicon, plastics—were put to miraculous new civilian uses.

In 1960, the year our family moved into the Techbuilt, a young kidney doctor in Seattle, experimenting with a slippery plastic called Teflon, created a nonclotting U-shaped shunt that could be left permanently in a patient's vein, thus turning dialysis—a wartime invention—from an emergency lifesaver into a routine though expensive and debilitating treatment. The same year, a trio of doctors and researchers at Johns Hopkins Hospital in Baltimore announced in the *Journal of the American Medical Association* that they had successfully restarted hearts that stopped beating under anesthesia by pressing rhythmically and repeatedly on the breastbone, thus paving the way for widespread use of cardiopulmonary resuscitation, or CPR.

We were in the midst of a revolution in medicine, one qualitatively different from any that had come before. The easy battles had been won. The mass conquests of microbes and viruses were mostly behind us. In their ongoing war against death, doctors were turning to new frontiers: the repair, restarting, and even replacement of human organs once considered sacred, vital, and inviolable.

One epicenter of the new revolution in medicine was Peter Bent Brigham Hospital, one of Harvard Medical School's flagship teaching and research institutions, located not far from my father's office in Boston's Back Bay. There, under the leadership of an aristocratic and charismatic chief of surgery named Francis Daniels Moore (who later became my mother's breast-cancer surgeon and possibly saved her life), doctors spent the mid-twentieth century in an orchestrated frenzy of daring human experimentation. Some surgeons used sterilized Dacron cut from used boat sails to patch ballooning aneurysms that threatened to fatally burst the walls of weak aortas, the giant arteries that carry red, oxygenated blood from the heart to smaller blood vessels throughout the body. Others, in the days before the phenomenon of organ rejection was understood, carried out experiments—almost all of them unsuccessful—in kidney transplantation.

The pioneering heart surgeon Dwight Harken drew on the

experience he'd gained in the summer of 1944 (as other doctors were saving my father's life in Italy), when he pulled shrapnel from the pulsing hearts of more than a hundred wounded
soldiers in England, breaking a long-standing medical taboo
against surgically invading the heart. At the Brigham in peacetime he went further, using his fingers and crude crochet-hook-
like tools to break open the stiff, scarred mitral heart valves
of young women condemned to invalidism and early death by
childhood rheumatic fever, a then-commonplace inflammation
of the heart caused by strep infections before the use of antibiotics was widespread. Harken's statistics were dismal at first: six
out of ten of his first heart-valve patients died on his Brigham
operating table or soon afterward. Among those who died were
some who could have lived restricted lives for years without surgery. But as techniques improved, Harken saved many lives.

In other operating rooms at the Brigham, early results were
equally grim, as surgeons cut out some patients' adrenal glands
in a futile effort to control their dangerously high blood pressure
and performed brain surgeries to remove the pituitary glands
from women with metastasized breast cancer in hopes of slowing its spread. (The women were left with brain damage on top
of their still-fatal illnesses.) In time, of course, the experiments
led to amazing victories: immune-suppressing drugs were discovered, kidney transplants saved thousands of lives, and survival rates for all sorts of surgeries improved radically as a result
of Francis Moore's research. But at a cost.

The Brigham's Harvard faculty doctors were well-educated,
often upper-class men like Moore; their patient-subjects were
mostly working-class Italian-Americans and Irish-Americans from
South and North Boston getting the charity care that the hospital had been founded to provide. There were no guidelines then
for experiments on human subjects, and some patients quietly
complained to the anthropologist Renée Fox that they had been

oversold on the potential benefits of their surgeries, and underinformed of their considerable risks. Some young doctors refused to participate altogether in what they called "murders" at the Brigham. A specialist in medical ethics warned against the "triumphalist temptation to slash and suture our way to eternal life."

But the experiments continued nonetheless, cheered on by an enthusiastic popular press. In 1963—a year before my father got the job he loved at Wesleyan and moved our rootless family, for the final time, to Middletown—*Time* magazine put Moore on its cover as a symbol of the bold, new medical era, celebrating his extensive research into making surgery safer. "With their new machines and new skills, surgeons know practically no limits to the range of patients they can help," the *Time* story read. It did not mention that that year, all nine Brigham patients who received experimental liver transplants died prolonged and horrible deaths, or that Moore had quietly ordered the transplants abandoned.

Moore later called that time "the black years," but never publicly disavowed the work he and others had done. "The patients selected were going to die shortly," he wrote of the first kidney transplantations, "[and] this experiment was being undertaken under the most ideal and favorable circumstances, with conscientious recording of every detail. Whatever criticism we have endured regarding the ethics of these early efforts as viewed in terms of present-day mores 40 years later, the fact is that if nothing is ventured, nothing is won." Moore's statement represented a revolution in attitudes toward the fatally ill: they were no longer souls in transition but experimental subjects whose medically prolonged suffering was justified by the hope of advancing scientific knowledge for the benefit of future patients.

Dwight Harken was among many Brigham doctors who looked back on the early deaths with something close to horror. When one of his early heart patients died, Harken said the pain he felt was "different than the pain of losing one's patient under standard circumstances. . . . then somehow we blame fate, the Creator, or the disease with that failure. But when we've created the vehicle of death, the bridge to destruction for our patient, that's another kind of pain—the pain of the pioneer."

Meanwhile, in the operating rooms of Variety Club Heart Hospital in Minneapolis, Minnesota, a daring young surgeon named Walt Lillehei was conducting experiments of his own. Sometimes described as the "father of open-heart surgery," Lillehei spent the 1950s specializing in so-called "blue babies"—listless children with clubbed fingers and a blue tinge to their skins, otherwise doomed to early deaths by congenital holes between the chambers of their hearts that allowed red oxygenated and blue deoxygenated blood to intermix. Lillehei would cool the child's body in a metal cattle-feeding trough filled with ice, inducing a physical state similar to hibernation, and then stop the heart with a direct injection of potassium chloride, one of three drugs conventionally used to execute convicts in the death chamber. While a newly invented heart-lung machine (essentially a sophisticated pump that ran the blood through coils of glass and plastic tubing to an oxygenating aerator) did the work of the child's heart and lungs, Lillehei stitched up the hole between the chambers. Then the child's body was warmed in a trough filled with warm water, and the heart restarted with a single shock from another new electrical device called a defibrillator. The luckiest children went on to live long, normal lives.

Often, though, Lillehei's surgical suturing damaged the tiny hearts' delicate nerve and conduction systems so that they could no longer maintain normal beats. In one particularly bad run of surgical experimentation, seven in a row of Lillehei's "blue babies" died this way. Some of the families were too poor to pay for gravestones. Lillehei was desperate. He turned to a young inventor named Earl Bakken, who had recently cofounded with his brother-in-law a small business called Medtronic to repair electronic machines for the research labs of local hospitals, including the University of Minnesota Medical School. Earl Bakken had been fascinated with electricity since seeing the movie *Frankenstein* when he was a child growing up poor in rural Minnesota. In the early thirties, around the same time that my naughty father was nearly blowing his fingers off in South Africa with homemade bombs, Bakken was tinkering in his family's basement workshop in Minnesota, cobbling together a functioning telephone system, a crude rotary mower, a robot that smoked cigarettes, firecrackers he could set off by remote control, and a rudimentary but nastily effective taser.

In January 1958, in a converted garage in Minneapolis heated by a potbellied stove—six years after the Grass Physiological Stimulator pulled R.A. back from the brink of death at Beth Israel Hospital in Boston—Bakken created the world's first fully portable electronic pacemaker. The main components were an off-the-shelf nine-volt rechargeable nickel-cadmium battery, two dials, a red light that blinked on and off, and two simple transistors that delivered a timed electrical pulse. Etched on newly invented silicon wafers, the transistors were based on a blueprint for an electronic metronome that Bakken found in *Popular Electronics*. His pacemaker, a giant advance over the Grass Physiologic Stimulator, was the love child of two postwar technological revolutions—one in cardiac surgery and another in miniaturizing electronics.

The first patient to get Bakken's Medtronic 5800 was a six-year-old girl with a congenital heart defect who had just undergone open-heart surgery. It hung from her neck like a heavy, old-fashioned press camera, with two wires inserted close to her heart through her chest wall. The wires repeatedly cued her heart with a tiny electrical spark until it recovered enough to resume beating on its own. Compared with the massive, full-body shocks of the Stimulator, the Medtronic 5800 was a breakthrough. But its wiring caused susceptibility to infection where it entered the body. Like the Stimulator, it was still a "bridge" technology—a clumsy device suitable mostly for helping patients to climb over a period of temporary organ failure.

In the fall of 1958, at the Karolinska Institute just north of Stockholm, an inventor named Rune Elmqvist and a surgeon named Åke Senning took the next leap. After months of experiments on dogs, the pair embedded a pacemaker and all of its wiring completely inside the human body for the first time. Their first patient was Arne Larsson, a desperately ill forty-three-year-old owner of a Swedish marine electronics firm. He'd been an avid ice-skater, golfer, and businessman until a viral infection, perhaps hepatitis contracted from eating tainted oysters, severely damaged his heart and liver. His heart kept up a slow and irregular twenty-eight beats per minute, and he fainted multiple times a day. His doctors thought his death was imminent. After repeated entreaties from Larsson's wife Else-Marie, the doctor and the inventor set aside their canine experiments long enough to try to save the man's life, though they felt the experiment was premature.

Elmqvist, the director of research for a budding Swedish electronics firm called Elema-Schönander, cleaned out a Kiwi shoe-polish tin and, using the tin as a mold, wedged in two small, rechargeable nickel-cadmium batteries, miscellaneous wiring, and two standard circuits etched on wafers of silicon. He filled the tin with medical-grade epoxy resin. Once the resin hardened, he pulled the contraption out of the tin. It looked like something from a garage workshop: a small, translucent hockey puck filled with coiled wires, a battery, and electronic odds and ends, trailing two stainless steel wires encapsulated in polyethylene sleeves. In one of the institute's operating rooms, Senning opened Larsson's chest and sewed the two wires along the outer surface of his heart. The puck-shaped generator was tucked into a pocket of skin in Larsson's abdomen. Larsson came out from surgery with a normal heartbeat. About six hours later, acid from the battery leaked into the casing and shorted out the pacemaker. Larsson went back into surgery and was given another one, which lasted a few weeks, only to be replaced by still another, this one longer lasting. With little further ado, Arne Larsson went back to skating, playing golf, and running his electronics business.

The pace of medical lifesaving was moving so quickly on so many fronts simultaneously that it soon required a new kind of hospital room: the intensive care unit (ICU). In Kansas City, Kansas, in 1961, a Dr. Robert Potter took over an open ward formerly used to nurse the county's impoverished elderly and set up eleven cubicles equipped with all the latest machinery and electronic monitors. Staffed by nurses and doctors fully trained in the lifesaving new practice of CPR, the ICU put all the new machines in one place.

Primitive respirators based on the design of vacuum cleaners used flexible plastic hoses to funnel blasts of air down the throats and into the failing lungs of people temporarily too sick or paralyzed to breathe on their own. The nation's first "crash carts," manufactured in Potter's father's sheet-metal shop, held all the new equipment, all the better to rush it to the bedside. There were endotracheal tubes to attach the new respirators to the throats of patients; "Ambu bags" that doctors could inflate and deflate by hand to temporarily deliver air; metal external defibrillator paddles to jolt the heart back to life; and bed boards to slip under the body, providing the firm surface needed for an external heart massage so vigorous that it often cracked ribs.

Patients poured in. In 1969 in Miami, for the first time, a man who'd dropped dead of a heart attack was successfully resuscitated by a combination of outside-the-hospital defibrillation and CPR. Victims of car accidents on the new federal superhighways were soon being sped to freshly built emergency rooms and ICUs throughout the United States, ferried in ambulances manned by newly certified emergency medical technicians, dispatched via the brand-new 911 system, established nationally in 1971. The driving force behind it all was President Lyndon B. Johnson, who'd barely survived a heart attack himself in 1955 in Middleburg, Virginia, and had been rushed to a naval hospital in a hearse doing double duty as an ambulance.

The 911 system and the new ICUs saved the lives of many otherwise hardy people in their primes who'd suffered a heart attack, overdosed on drugs, been in a head-on collision, drowned, or been stabbed, shot, or accidentally poisoned. At the same time, the units obliterated Western death rituals, reshaped the architecture of the hospital, transformed the meaning of the body, and brutally deformed the way families, doctors, nurses—and even the dying themselves—behaved at the deathbed.

In the nineteenth century, dying usually meant waiting. In "The Sisters," set in 1895, James Joyce described such a vigil for a sixty-five-year-old priest dying in a poor Dublin parish:

There was no hope for him this time: it was the third stroke. Night after night I had passed the house (it was vacation time) and studied the lighted square of window: and night after night I had found it lighted in the same way, faintly and evenly. If he was dead, I thought, I would see the reflection of candles on the darkened blind for I knew that two candles must be set at the head of a corpse. He had often said to me, "I am not long for this world," and I had thought his words idle. Now I knew they were true.

A fellow priest received the dying man's final confession, anointed his forehead with oil, and spoke the litany of ancient Latin phrases marking the universal passage from life to death. When it was over, the priest's two sisters washed their brother's body and dressed him for his coffin.

In the metallic, machine-filled ICU, where death was fought to a standstill and its arrival regarded as an emblem of medical failure, such sacred rites of passage all but disappeared. Nurses often looked first at the monitors and then at the patient. The dying person was no longer in charge of his or her own death: doctors were the new authorities, and they popped in and out on rounds. There were technical specialists to treat each discrete bodily organ but nobody to minister to the emotional or spiritual needs of the dying person or the family. Latin liturgy gave way to talk of blood gases. Busyness supplanted waiting. Family members who once kept the death vigil, wiped the brows of the dying, changed their bedclothes, and listened to their last words were restricted to visiting hours. Months after the experience, family members, especially those who took part in decisions to remove people they loved from life support, experienced high rates of anxiety, depression, and symptoms of post-traumatic stress disorder. Often there were no "last words" because the mouths of the dying were stopped by the tubes of respirators and their minds sunk in chemical twilights to keep them from tearing out the lines that bound them to earth.

The new machines ushered in a transformation in the meaning of the body. It was no longer the temple of the soul but a housing for organs to be removed, rejiggered, and replaced like spare parts. The heart—the mystical seat of wisdom, love, and courage; the telltale heart that could harden, break, soften, knock, and open; the heart that knew what the mind could not comprehend—was now a pump. The lungs were a bellows, the kidneys, a sieve.

As the up-to-the-minute machines spread to newly prosperous countries around the world, they transformed not only the meaning of the aging and dying body but also its look. "The number of plump corpses has been on the rise recently," wrote Shinmon Aoki in *Coffinman,* a memoir of his work as a Japanese Buddhist mortician in the 1980s:

> These plumped-up, celadon-colored bodies take on the appearance of water-filled plastic bags. When I first started out washing and coffining corpses early in 1965, the majority of cases were home deaths. I'd go to a farming home in the foothills to find a corpse with a withered frame like a dead tree. . . . They looked like dried-up shells, the chrysalis from which the cicada had fled.
>
> Along with the economic advances in our country, though, we no longer see these corpses that look like dead trees. . . . The corpses that leave the hospital are all plumped up, both arms blackened painfully by needle marks made at transfusion, some with catheters and tubes still dangling from throat or lower abdomen. . . . There's nothing natural about the way they die, as the image of dried leaves falling in late autumn would impart. This tells us that our medical facilities leave us no room to think of death.
>
> The dying patient is surrounded by medical staff who, with its life support systems, has only one thought in mind: to extend life as long as possible. Next is the family and relatives who think there's nothing more important than life. For the patients confronting death, they wait alone inside that cold equipment on a stage prepared to struggle against death. But even if they wanted to prepare themselves for death, there's no one to give them advice, and

in that state they die. Even if they wanted to talk it over with someone, there only returns the litany of "Gambatte!" ("Hang in there!").

Not all doctors and nurses were pleased with the changes, and few other developed countries embraced medical technology with quite the gusto of the United States. Fewer ICUs—and far fewer dialysis units, for that matter—were established in my old home country, Britain, where funding decisions were made by regional administrators for the money-pinched and budget-conscious National Health Service. They faced other claims on their resources, such as paying the salaries of doctors to provide good, universal, free primary care, and even employing geriatric psychiatrists who, as late as the 1990s, made house calls. The British medical system now costs about half as much as does that of the United States, but its citizens have better overall health.

A decade after the first intensive care and coronary care units were established in England, a study in the *Lancet* found that the new units—whose beeping electronic machines terrified some patients—conferred "no clear advantage" over home care for heart-attack victims. Another study, published in the *British Medical Journal,* found in 1976 that patients over sixty and those suffering a first, uncomplicated heart attack did slightly better at home. Today, about 2 percent of beds in British hospitals are intensive care beds; in the United States, the figure is more than 11 percent. As a consequence of their relative scarcity, intensive care beds in Britain are less often the place where the elderly die.

In 1968, a decade after Arne Larsson's first pacemaker and sixteen years after Zoll saved R.A.'s life with the Physiological Stimulator, a pathologist named William St. Clair Symmers at Charing Cross Hospital in London described a troubling case, a harbinger of thousands more to come. Lifesaving machines were evolving so rapidly and scrambling moral and medical categories in such confusing ways that the soft technologies of clinical practice and common sense could not keep up. The unspoken maxim had become, "If we can, we must."

In a letter to the *British Medical Journal* entitled "Not Allowed to Die," Dr. Symmers described a retired sixty-eight-year-old doctor who'd been admitted to "an overseas hospital" (most likely in the United States) with stomach cancer that had fatally metastasized to his lymph, liver, and spine. After one surgery to remove much of his stomach and another to clear a blood clot from his lung, the dying doctor-patient asked that "no steps should be taken to prolong his life, for the pain of his cancer was now more than he would needlessly continue to endure. He himself wrote a note to this effect in his case records."

Two weeks later the desperately ill doctor had a heart attack while still in the hospital. Five times in a single night his heart stopped, and five times the emergency-resuscitation team rushed to his bedside and restarted it. Morning found the man in one of the ambiguous halfway states being created so frequently by life-support machines that new medical terms—such as *persistent vegetative state* and *brain death*—were being invented to describe them.

Resuscitation had kept alive his brain stem—the most primitive, reptilian part of the central nervous system—and it kept signaling his heart to beat and his lungs to rise and fall. But the folded rind of his neocortex, the advanced, thinking portion of his brain, was dead from lack of oxygen. Gone was what we commonly call the "self," the personality, or even the soul. The man's body was still pink. The skin cells in his earlobes, fingers, and toes still absorbed oxygen and nutrients, and expelled waste products. His lungs moved in and out, and his beating heart still pumped blood and oxygen to cells throughout his body. But he could not easily be described as either living or dead. He had clenched, turned-in hands and could not speak or move or respond to sound. The tools of modern lifesaving had forced upon him the sufferings of life without its joys, and the helplessness of death without its peace.

What was left of the doctor lingered for three weeks, experiencing seizures and projectile vomiting. Doctors and nurses fed him intravenously, gave him blood transfusions, administered antibiotics to ward off pneumonia, and cut a hole in his windpipe to keep his airway clear. The man's heart stopped for the last time as the hospital team prepared to attach him to a respirator. "This case report is submitted for publication without commentary or conclusions," wrote Dr. Symmers, "which are left for those who may read it to provide for themselves. . . . The identity of those concerned and of their country is beside the point."

My parents, like most people outside the field of medicine, were virtually oblivious to the moral quandaries arising, beyond the little that surfaced in an occasional issue of *Time* or *Life*. They were in their forties in the late 1960s, youthful and healthy, recently arrived at Wesleyan, and busy with other things, such as making new friends, building another Techbuilt, and establishing themselves in Middletown. My mother was in a graduate program, earning a master of arts in teaching. I was a junior at Wesleyan, studying Shakespeare and Virginia Woolf and living off-campus. My brother Michael was at an experimental boarding school in upstate New York, and Jonathan was struggling through a local boys' Catholic high school, serving as coxswain for a crew club he'd organized on the Connecticut River and fixing cars in his spare time.

In the fall of 1970, when my mother was forty-seven and teaching art at Deep River High School, the surgical advances pioneered at the Brigham by Francis Daniels Moore may well have saved her life. She found a lump in her left breast. At Middlesex Hospital, she was given a radical mastectomy, the drastic surgical approach then in fashion. The surgeon removed her breast, much of the muscle of her left chest wall, a hard cancerous tumor the size of a walnut, and four cancerous lymph nodes, including one totally eclipsed by a metastasized second tumor. This was a sign that cancer cells had drifted through her lymph fluid and might have spread elsewhere in her body. After six months of grueling radiation treatments, she drove with my father to Boston to meet with Dr. Moore at the Brigham. She was worried about a recurrence.

Francis Daniels Moore was fifty-eight then and still the Brigham's chief of surgery. Gray-haired and upright, he counted advanced breast cancer among his many fields of expertise. He was aware, as was my mother, of the risks she faced. As he later wrote in his autobiography, "The stark reality is that almost all patients who enter this wilderness of advanced disease [that is, a recurrence after an initial treatment for breast cancer] will die." He took substantial time with her, examined her lumpy but noncancerous remaining breast, and advised her to have it removed as well, to be on the safe side. She took his advice and survived the simple mastectomy he performed. Her cancer never returned.

She had no regrets about sacrificing her breasts for a shot at saving her life. She was grateful to Moore and to her cancer support group and to her radiation techs for her survival—as well as to her own formidable life force. But cancer changed her. She read Aleksandr Solzhenitsyn's *Cancer Ward* and Elizabeth Kübler-Ross's 1969 bestseller, *On Death and Dying*. She looked her own death in the face.

She photographed herself naked, her scarred and bony chest exposed to her Nikkormat camera. She developed the negatives in the darkroom my father had built her, made a few prints, showed nobody, and filed them carefully away along with the contact sheets. She put up her blond-streaked hair in her signature

French twist just as she'd always done, continued to dress impec-
cably, and went out into the world as the beautiful woman she'd
always been. She never had reconstructive surgery, and after a few
years she stopped tucking her sloshy, saline-filled replacement
boobs into her bra, and lived instead as a flat-chested woman.

Instead of returning to teaching art, she ferried more than
one faculty wife stricken by cancer to her chemotherapy
appointments and helped shepherd them and other women to
their deaths. She was glad to be alive, among the lucky ones,
but the more she saw of American medicine poised at the brink
of death, the more she questioned its tendency to overreach. In
1977, as she was emerging psychically from the shadow of her
own cancer, she spent time with a divorced faculty wife named
Bolly Hassan, who had pancreatic cancer, one of the disease's
deadliest forms. Bolly was given a surgery called the Whipple
procedure, an eviscerating, last-ditch approach far more radical than my mother's radical mastectomy, more damaging to
the quality of a patient's remaining life, and with real but slim
chances of prolonged success. The Whipple removed the cancerous head of Bolly's pancreas, her entire gall bladder, and a
portion of her small intestine and stomach. What was left of her
internal organs was reconnected to her remaining large intestine. It didn't work. As Bolly lay dying in the hospital, skin and
bones and barely conscious, a nurse came in once a day to move
her body to a bedside scale for weighing, a pointless operation
that made Bolly whimper, until my mother said to the nurse,
"She's dying! Can't you see she's in pain?" and insisted she stop.

My mother's disquiet was not unique. The new technologies
seemed to have blunted medical staff to the suffering their procedures caused the dying, and often postponed death without
restoring health. They created unrealistic hopes of immortality
in some doctors and patients and bred a toxic mistrust between
them that persists to this day. They helped produce doctors of

great technical prowess and limited training in emotional communication. And they brought to light a lack of cultural consensus about the doctor's evolving moral role near the end of life.

From the plagues of the Black Death during the Middle Ages through the epidemics of typhoid, cholera, scarlet fever, and tuberculosis that blighted later centuries, doctors, like their patients, moved through a world of random, widespread, and premature death. They understood death as a given throughout the life span. There was usually little they could do except suggest remedies such as port wine, bloodletting, and mercury. So they sat with the dying in their suffering, predicted the coming of the final crises, and waited. They accepted the natural course of events.

After the mid-1950s, the attitudes of many doctors and patients shifted from faith in God and acceptance of death to faith in medicine and resistance of death. There was always *something,* no matter how ultimately futile, that a doctor or nurse could do.

Patients weren't always grateful. In a small rural hospital in Virginia in the mid-1970s, a nurse came proudly to the bed of an elderly woman whose life she'd saved by performing a cardiopulmonary resuscitation that had cracked two of the old woman's ribs. "I will hate you till the day I die," the old woman said. "You took away my chance to go to heaven, and on top of that you hurt me."

In 1977, the year Bolly Hassan died, a young doctor named Diane Meier—who would later become a MacArthur fellow and a leader of the medical countermovement known as palliative care—was studying medicine at an Oregon Health & Science University hospital in Portland, Oregon. On her first day as an intern, Meier was part of a medical team that subjected an eighty-nine-year-old man dying of heart failure to a series of violent and ultimately unsuccessful resuscitations.

"The fundamental principles that had guided the practice of medicine—relieve suffering, do no harm—were upended," Meier wrote years later:

> Almost without discussion, the primary moral principle underlying medical practice became the obligation to prolong life regardless of the toll in suffering, poor quality of life, or cost.
>
> Other messages, equally powerful and similarly unstated, were conveyed when no one on the team stopped to speak with the patient's eighty-seven-year-old wife after he died; no one asked me how I was handling this violent death of one of my patients on my first day as a real doctor.

CHAPTER 6

MY FATHER'S OPEN HEART

My parents soldiered on across a rough plateau, with no outside caregiving help beyond Annie, who still gave my father his showers. The unintended consequences of my father's pacemaker did not show themselves at once. He came back to Pine Street from Middlesex hospital in January of 2003 with his hernias fixed, his pacemaker ticking, his death forestalled, and his brain just a little bit worse. A man in his forties or fifties might have bounced back from the two minor surgeries with ease, but not my eighty-year-old father: general anesthesia can be stressful on the aged brain, and studies suggest that somewhere between 6 and 30 percent of the elderly suffer at least a temporary decline in cognitive functioning afterward. My mother noticed that my father had more trouble finding words, couldn't follow movie plots, went repeatedly to the wall calendar in the kitchen to check the day's appointments, and obsessed about the investments he no longer controlled. Once he worriedly told me to "call the police" when my mother was fifteen minutes late in returning from a lunch date. On a walk we took to one of our favorite spots, Indian Hill Cemetery, he seemed strangely drawn to an arrangement of nails on the crossbar of a gate, pointing them out to me as if they had a significance that I could not fathom.

Alarmed, my mother took him to his neurologist, who called it a temporary "slippage" and a "mild decompensation," probably attributable to the surgeries. Medicare authorized more speech therapy, and the dedicated and perceptive Angela returned to the house three times a week.

When Annie left town due to a family emergency, my mother again collapsed into tears and exhaustion. She and I were falling into what would become a pattern: my father would get worse, I'd nag her to get more help, and she'd resist until she hit the wall. Then I'd fly in, and she'd become, as my brother Michael put it, "sweetly reasonable" and agree to a change. But this time I had a work deadline and didn't want to go.

It had taken me more than a year to realize that my brothers weren't carrying much of the load. Charming, creative, and often financially struggling middle-aged men whom my mother and I still called "the boys," they had not visited Middletown once in the year since the stroke, although they had taken to calling more frequently, and my brother Jonathan often lent me a listening ear during his long hours on the road.

In part, my mother and I could blame only ourselves: neither of us had asked for nor expected much from them. This had a perverse payoff for me. After decades of secretly fearing that my mother's accusations of selfishness were true, I was, at last, her Good Daughter. During one of my visits, as I was explaining her investments to her for the *nth* time, she sighed and said, "Thank God I have a daughter. Sons are useless." That felt, in a strange way, bad, and in a strange way, good.

I pressured Jonathan to fly to Connecticut, and he did. A practical fixer, he negotiated a good deal for our mother on a new Camry and took her to buy a cell phone in hopes that it would release her to hire someone to look after our father and yet be reachable if something went wrong. In honor of their shared love of sailing, he took our dad to Mystic Seaport for a day, to walk around the old schooners and whaling ships. My father tired quickly, could not carry on a conversation, and asked to go home early. Jonathan gave up on him for good.

"In retrospect, it was selfish on my part," Jonathan would tell me later, looking back. "He wasn't the guy I was used to, and I didn't feel like being a babysitter. Now I tell my friends, spend all the time you can with them. It'll make you feel better later."

My mother returned the cell phone the day Jonathan flew out, infuriating her by failing to strip the linens from his bed. My heart sank. Neither he nor I was sure the trip had been worth it.

One night, when I was out of ideas, Jonathan called me from the road—his new job involved driving big rigs around Los Angeles, working punishing hours for not much more than minimum wage—to say, "I think I've pulled a rabbit out of a hat." He'd given our exhausted mother the phone number of a friend named Toni Perez-Palma who needed part-time work and was living in Meriden, a deindustrialized city near Middletown that had once been famous for manufacturing tools and silver cutlery. Jonathan first met Toni years earlier, when she was traveling the country with one of his truck driver friends. She and Jonathan bonded over their mutual commitment to recovery from addiction, and they stayed in touch.

On the day Toni first drove her battered SUV up my parents' long drive, guided in from the street by my anxious, mute father, my mother knew little about her, and what little she knew did not reassure her. The nervousness ran both ways. "Your mother was sitting at the dining room table with a big legal pad in front of her," Toni later told me. "I was intimidated by her proper British air. When she opened her mouth with that accent, I was afraid I was going to blurt out some slur."

My mother asked Toni if she'd ever done this kind of work before. My father hovered in the background, pacing. Toni thought he had a sweet presence and liked his smile. The good-looking daughter of Puerto Rican and Italian immigrants, Toni had grown up mainly in foster care and dropped out of school in tenth grade. After some lost years knocking around Miami, she'd changed her life, gone to work as a waitress and a bartender, managed a restaurant, and earned her GED. She was five years clean and sober by the time she met my mother, and she hoped someday to get a degree in geriatric social work. She was caring for her own aged biological mother, worrying about her two grown kids, and taking medication for a chronic condition that restricted her from working more than a few hours a week.

She did not tell my mother all this, not right away. Instead she described the work she'd done earlier helping her mother take care of elderly people in Miami. Toni was strong, patient, honest, and energetic. She loved old people and she had a big heart. My mother was desperate. And Toni was a gift from unseen powers.

Soon she was my mother's right hand, driving her SUV up the driveway three times a week, giving my father his morning shower, blow-drying his hair, cleaning up breakfast, vacuuming, and doing the emotional and physical work that I, had I been a different daughter, might have taken up. My mother often worked alongside her, and together they weeded the garden, stained the deck, and squirted a perimeter of poison around the house each spring to keep out the ants.

The healing went both ways. "I was pleased to have a job," Toni told me later. "I felt useful. It was good for my self-esteem. And the more duties I started to do, the more duties she gave me, and I got a relationship with both of them where I was not just an employee but also a friend."

And so she became one of two and a half million street saints across the country who, despite poor pay and the harshness of their own lives, draw on unseen wells of compassion and emotional skill for families like mine. My mother paid into Social Security for her and, in time, came to pay her nearly twice the immorally low going rate. But Toni was not federally entitled to the minimum wage or overtime pay or any other basic protection of the Fair Labor Standards Act, on the theory that workers like her—most of them women—are near-family members who mainly provide companionship and therefore, in a logic that escapes me, don't deserve decent pay. In a further reflection of our culture's willingness to pay millions for high-tech "cures" (usually provided by men) but very little for ongoing care (usually provided by women), repeated attempts to cover home workers under federal labor laws have run into resistance since the 1930s and into the first decade of the twenty-first century; the home-health agencies that employ many of them have recently been prime lobbyists against change.

It was Toni who rinsed and dried the lettuce and wrapped it in dish towels for the refrigerator crisper, the way my mother liked it. It was she who called my father "Mr. Butler," even as she quietly set aside his shit-stained bathrobe for the wash. She was not a servant, not exactly a hired hand, and not quite a surrogate daughter, and yet she was a bit of all those things. She kept my mother out of the grave and my father out of a nursing home. She probably did as much good for my father and mother as all their children combined and more than most of their doctors. She sometimes felt more like a sister to me than my brothers felt like brothers.

She was patient and kind to my father in a way my frayed mother could not be and tolerant of my mother in ways that I was not. "Your mother had very little patience because she had waited so long to accept help," Toni explained to me some time later. "She was sleep deprived, and she was there all the time, so no wonder she got impatient. And your father, he had a demeanor of sweetness. He was easy, he was like—he was not my child—he was something more than a job—he was something more special."

I kept doing what I thought I did best and what I thought I would be loved for: I played social worker, found experts, nagged, bossed, strategized, and planned for the worst. But maybe the best thing I did was write my father love letters.

They were simple letters, as if written by a five-year-old girl. Knowing that his visual brain was less damaged than his language centers, I put drawings in the margins and within the text. My drawings were little cartoons, imperfect, sloppy; my handwriting as hard to read as ever. I no longer had to worry about how he'd edit my work or what he'd say about my risky career. He wrote back more tenderly than he could speak. It was the laboring-over that counted for me, the fact that he'd spent an afternoon making something, a gift, for me.

For decades we'd had such high standards for each other, and never hesitated to make it clear when the other one hadn't met them. In my teenage years I'd wanted him to drink and flirt less at parties, to pay more attention to my brothers, to stand up to my mother and protect me from her, and to be more encouraging and attentive of me. He'd wanted me to do my homework, to stop losing things, to stop fighting with my mother, to

stop contradicting him at the dinner table, and to live up to my
"potential." Now he looked at me with fresh eyes, impressed
when, after a walk with him through the Wadsworth Woods, I
did something perfectly ordinary like scrape mud off my shoes
before getting back into the car. And I, in turn, marveled at his
ability to walk down to the Wesleyan pool all by himself.

Perhaps it would have been better for my mother if my father
had died of his stroke, and perhaps it would have been better
for him. But it wouldn't have been better for me. His aphasia
unlocked my tongue and my father's heart. In an outpouring of
love and gratitude, I thanked him for all he had done for me, and
I got back nothing but love in return. Perhaps I was intuitively
preparing for his death.

I did not write to him about the fact that in my memory I
have two different fathers: the loving, exciting one of my early
English childhood, and the remote, overworked, irascible,
intimidating lion who dominated our dinner table in the United
States. I didn't write about his drawing me into endless intellectual arguments, or the barrage of accusations—*you drive me
to drink, you're sick in the head*—that I heard when I fought
with my mother, stayed out too late with boys, or was labeled
an underachiever. I said nothing about the day on the lake in
Wellesley when he slapped me hard in the face while trying to
teach me to sail, nor about the many mornings he yelled at me
at the breakfast table until I went off to catch the school bus
late and in tears, sure that I was no longer loved.

I wrote about him reading me *Babar the Elephant*.

In what I came to think of as "legacy letters," I thanked him for
lending me money to buy my first San Francisco house, and for:

not giving up on me through years of conflict, for opening
your heart to me now. It is wonderful to live my life knowing
I have my father's blessing. All of this will stay with me until

I die. It has formed me in ways I don't even know. You communicated your enjoyment of this complicated and often painful life we are given—just as I saw it when you marched around the house conducting your invisible orchestras. These things are in my bones, in my muscles, in my cells, and when I think of you I know that these are among the gifts you have given me. Thank you for my love of life.

The little girl whose father stroked her face. The little girl standing on top of her father's shoulders and jumping into the sea. The years of fighting and pain and estrangement. And through it all, a strong cord of love that connects me to you and will never be broken.

My father wrote back. "It is difficult for me to express the love I feel for you, but you seem to know it deeply. How can I end a letter that expresses such joy? All I can do is say thank you."

Urged on by Angela and encouraged by a Wesleyan student who came every week to coach him on the computer, my father struggled to write his autobiography. It was called "Recall," a single-spaced four-page recitation of his South African boyhood and his wounding in Italy during the Second World War. It took him months.

"As a boy, I constantly ran into trouble, mostly of a physical kind," the autobiography began. "I was incapable of staying away from danger." Following a familiar litany of his boyhood scrapes in the South African desert, such as burning his leg in a smoldering garbage pit while looking for car batteries containing lead for his father's linotypes, he described his first serious brush with death. When he was fifteen, he and a boarding-school friend named Jack Osborne, a boy from Rhodesia who was staying with him over the Christmas holidays, made plans to go joyriding with other boys by "borrowing" one of the cars parked in a Cradock garage while the car's owners were at the movies. My father and Jack were late to the rendezvous because Jack spent hours at the house of a girl he was courting, listening to her play the piano while my father waited, agonized, on the porch. Finally Jack said his good-byes and the two of them rushed to the garage just in time to see the two red taillights of the fatal car, loaded with my father's cousins and other friends, disappear around a bend and speed toward the National Road. It was going about seventy miles an hour across the desert floor when it hit an unlit donkey cart and catapulted upside down into a ditch. Two young cousins, white-faced, ran the two miles back to the town police station. Flung out of the car into the veld were the dying bodies of two of my father's closest friends, one of them the son of the garage owner. A third boy survived with brain damage so severe that he could never return to school.

I put down the text. My father had told me this story so often that I could see it in my mind's eye: the girl playing piano in a pool of light; my father pacing the porch; he and Jack Osborne racing through the dusty streets to the garage in the desert night, running after two red taillights—and here my father would sweep out his hand—chasing death and failing to catch it.

I picked up "Recall" again. Next my father described the turning point of his life, his near-fatal wounding in Italy. "The war was increasing in ferocity," the section opened:

My platoon was involved from daybreak and I was set up to go on a patrol and to take the village of Panzano. With a Bren gun I had to cover a small group of my comrades. Enemy infantry soon tackled them. Firing became general. A mortar bomb went right into the hole I was sheltering in and exploded with real effect. This changed the nature of the fight. My first reaction was to find my gun, which I did a few yards away. Then I became aware of blood oozing onto the ground. It took me some time to realize that the blood was all mine.

Like an idiot—or a daughter in a state of denial—I marked up the text, suggested improvements, and sent it back to him as if he were still the man he'd once been. When my mother called and gently and tenderly told me, "He needs encouragement," I understood how far wrong I'd gone.

And still our love went on, poured from imperfect and broken vessels. It was my parents' custom, every September, to exchange birthday notes to each other, and neither the stroke or the pacemaker, nor my father's decline, changed that. On the morning of September 16, 2003, my father left a short note at their breakfast table commemorating my mother's seventy-ninth birthday, a note he'd labored over the night before:

My Dear,

It is past midnight or rather where midnight ought to be. We are right into your birthday.

How can I give you adequate thanks for all you have done for me?

It is not possible and I must simply say I can't.

This note simply says you have given me all the help I need.

All my love,

Jeff

Nine days later, my mother pulled out her calligraphy pens and made three starts at a birthday letter to him.

"My Darling," one of them began:

Over the years you have written me beautiful letters for my birthdays. I can't match your elegance and tender expressions. I want you to know I love you for your sweet nature and patience with my frustrations with "life, as it is." You rarely, if ever, complain about your difficulties, and sometimes I wish you would to make me feel better about my complaining!

On another sheet, my mother copied out the final stanza of a poem written by my father's brother Guy in the summer of 1944, the year my father's left arm was blown to tatters in Italy:

To Any Young Soldier

. . . So light a fag, knock back a glass or two
Look calmly on shell torn terraces,
All last night's acre of especial hell;
And wonder if the years ahead of you
Will stretch like kilo-stones or cypresses
From eighteen on to eighty, or the next shell.

"Well, it was the next shell," my mother wrote. "And here we are together at eighty after all that you have gone through with calm acceptance. Thank you for our life together, and for being so patient living with a difficult woman for fifty-plus years. Happy eighty-first—Hang in there—we'll make it together. Love, Val."

If only he had died that year.

III

ORDEAL

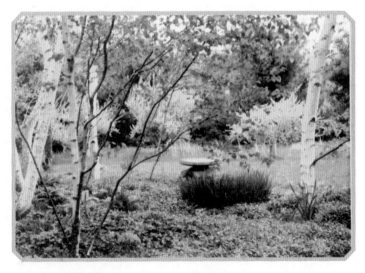

Autumn at Pine Street, Middletown, Connecticut.

CHAPTER 7

NOT GETTING BETTER

In October of 2003, my mother went to a stationery store and bought a blank-lined book with a stiff, sea-green cloth cover. It was Quakerish in its simplicity and would not have been out of place in my great-grandfather James Butler's newspaper office in turn-of-the-twentieth-century South Africa. On its first page, in her upright italic script, she wrote, "This is the social worker's idea, to sort out the thoughts that keep me anxious. I am not myself. At times I am overwhelmed by what I have to do." She was seventy-nine.

She was suffering from worsened insomnia and sleeping two and a half hours a night. She'd broken down in tears in the office of a new, hastily engaged (and, it turned out, not entirely competent) financial adviser, who'd referred her to a psychiatrist. The psychiatrist sent her on to a social worker and also prescribed Remeron, an antidepressant reputed to help with anorexia and sleeplessness. She was desperate enough to try it. Three years earlier she'd have refused it as a crutch for the cowardly and the weak.

She did not write a word in her journal about my father's condition, nor did she tell me about the increasingly troubling signs she'd seen of his further decline. He was having trouble remembering how to start the computer and open up Microsoft Word. After a urinary tract infection and a bout of bronchitis, he'd had an episode of confusion and had fallen three times in a single day.

She drew a line down the middle of a blank page and headed it "Retirement Place." Under *Pros,* she wrote four words: "Maintenance taken care of." *Cons* filled the right side of the page: "*All* aged. Conservative Republicans! Intellectual Stimulation in Question. Communal Dining. Aesthetics! Space Limited. Even if we both go into an apartment Jeff would need constant help of some sort or another. It is not going to be without problems, which will show themselves later on. Nothing is 100 percent *ever.*"

Under "Staying Home—Pros," she listed "Less boring. More familiar surroundings. Own doctors. Near Middlesex Hospital. More space. Convenient location. Less expensive." Under *Cons:* "Maintenance is a big job."

She did not have a son nearby to make minor home repairs or change the light bulbs in her high-ceilinged vestibule, nor did she know a nice young man from church, since she had no church. Her own mother had lived independently into her nineties in a house two doors down from her devoted oldest son. But neither of my brothers was any more willing than I was to move back into a childhood bedroom and submit to her rigid mealtimes, unasked-for advice on diet, career, and grooming, dominion over the kitchen, and need for order and control.

The Remeron kicked in, and she started sleeping. Within a month, she stopped seeing the social worker and returned to her default setting: stoic, frugal self-reliance. Moment-to-moment caregiving had damaged her ability to think strategically and flexibly—never her strong suit in any case. "I feel so much better, more myself with the old energy," she wrote in her journal after she let the social worker go. "There are places in my life that still feel shut off and cramped by my circumstances," she went on. "I need to face plans for when things get worse—what if Jeff needs to go someplace to be looked after? *Where?* I also need more space for myself—away, alone, not caring for J. all the time. I miss that."

I drove her to western Massachusetts to check out one last old-age place: the cream of the crop, I'd been told, a retirement community with three levels of care, founded by retired professors from Amherst. A friend of mine had successfully placed her disabled sister there. The buildings were set among empty green hills and were overheated, spotless, and upholstered, like a nice Radisson. The vegetables at lunch were, as usual, overcooked; a van was available for trips to a small town somewhere out of sight; the apartments had wheelchair-accessible showers and no decks or doors opening to the natural world. I could not imagine my mother there. With my support, she decided to continue toughing things out at home. She would meet her future there when it came.

"I still feel like part of me is back in Connecticut with you," I wrote her after I got back to California.

This was a terribly important visit. I stopped being ambivalent, or resisting, or fearing the change in our relationship. I do not see helping you as a burden. I see it as a responsibility that is based in deep love, and therefore it brings joy and satisfaction. It is part of my own passage to adult life.

One morning you were in a panic and flying off the handle and for the first time, perhaps, I saw you with the eyes of compassion—I could *see* that you were afraid and overwhelmed—and my reactive fear and anger disappeared. Where do these gifts come from, these final growings-up?

I am honored to help you the best I can, the way you have helped me, darned my socks, put up my hems, and listened to me.

In November 2003, my father's speech therapy was stopped, and with it, his work on "Recall." Even though most of the sky-rocketing increase in Medicare costs is due to advanced and expensive medical technologies (such as pacemakers, defibrillators, heart-valve surgeries, chemotherapy, dialysis, and the like), Congress, in an attempt to cut costs, limited payments for hands-on speech and physical therapy that year to about $1,600 each. After an uproar from constituents, it suspended the limit—but reiterated Medicare's long-standing practice of providing coverage only while patients showed improvement, and not to keep them from slipping back. (To settle a class-action lawsuit, Medicare agreed to liberalize this practice in late 2012.) Medicare had spent roughly $30,000 on getting my father through his stroke, installing his pacemaker, and fixing his hernias. It paid about $7,300, all told, for his speech therapy, perhaps the greatest contributor to the quality of his extended life.

Angela, the speech therapist, generously continued to come without pay on Saturday mornings, inspired by my father's desire, she told me later, "to continue to work and improve himself against all odds." But she was pregnant with her first child, and in the spring of 2004, close to the end of her pregnancy, she had to stop. My father's computer coach begged off, too, after telling my mother that my father was forgetting everything he learned from week to week. My mother took over the computer, set up her own e-mail account (her pass code was Harpy1), and relegated my father to eking out his letters by hand. She put "Recall"—the last, unfinished flowering of his literary life—into a filing drawer. Toni watched with deep dismay and said nothing.

"He looked forward to the rapport with the young man, even if he didn't need to know anything more about the computer," Toni told me later. "If it was me, I'd have said, 'Do you mind coming for the hour anyway?' It was good for Jeff's emotional well-being. Your mother and I, we were caretakers, women, and this gave him a chance to be with another man. Your father stopped using the computer completely then—it was something that stimulated his mind, and your mother snatched it away from him. And then the autobiography stopped, and he left me in Siena, with blood running down him, and he didn't know his arm was blown off."

Neither my mother nor I had the wit to take "Recall" to a copy shop, make a little spiral-bound book of it, and arrange a reading for their friends. My mother was too busy taking care of my father, and perhaps too protective of his dignity to put him on display. I was too busy living my split life and trying to peer beyond the headlights into the dark landscape before us.

My father accepted what he could not change. But he paid a price. When my mother asked him one day whether he was depressed, he told her yes.

He was "living too long," he said.

She never told me this. But she did tell his neurologist, Dr. Margaret O'Donohue, and my father acknowledged to the doctor that he'd said it. Dr. O'Donohue wrote in her clinical notes that she wasn't sure if he still thought that way and tentatively suggested an antidepressant, but my parents seemed reluctant to explore it. Depressed, isolated people are more likely to fall prey to dementia, but I did not know that, and I wasn't in on the conversation in any case.

One morning in the kitchen, my father watched me unstacking the dishwasher. He said, "This house is full of things I used to do." There was a silence. He looked straight at me with a great vehemence and said, "I am *not* going to get better."

CHAPTER 8

DHARMA SISTERS

My father didn't just fail to get better. He got worse. The letters he wrote me grew shorter, the handwriting wobbly, the little faces in the text harder to make out, the lines increasingly speckled with cross-outs, strange repetitions, meaningless sentences, and odd word choices. One read, almost in its entirety:

> I wish I knew the precise shape this letter was going to take.
> I want to write as clearly as I can without messing around. . . .
> I have put pen to paper with dubious results. I am particularly
> upset that I am nowhere near the shape I want to be. I am having
> lots of trouble writing and your mother is understandably upset.

I felt my heart sink, but I did not linger on what this might imply. Another letter read, "You will notice that I am full of rhetoric most of the time, full of rhetoric in the most rhetorical way. It is very repetitive. But you do try."

On the last day of 2003, about a year after installation of the pacemaker, my father briefly lost most of his already limited capacity to speak, and my mother took him to the hospital for a new round of tests. The tests turned up nothing new except another urinary tract infection—a common cause of confusion in the elderly—and after some days his speech returned. They kept on keeping on: she took care of him and gardened and checked out videos from the public library. Together they watched *The Misfits, On the Waterfront,* and *Bridge over the River Kwai.* My father wrote me a few letters, more coherent ones, catching me up on news: he'd gotten $12,000 worth of dental implants. He'd watched the neighbors' grandchildren, visiting from England, try to retrieve a toy plane stuck in a tree. Ben Carton, a former student who was almost a surrogate son, had made his yearly visit with his young family. There'd been a visit from M'ellen Kennedy, one of Jonathan's former girlfriends, whom my mother had taken under her wing as a teenager and nicknamed Peaches. Another of my father's beloved former Wesleyan students, a financial wizard who'd retired early and earned her pilot's license, visited during commencement and brought my parents a bottle of wine.

There was more that my father did not, perhaps could not, tell me. One day, my mother said, he forgot his way home from the pool and wandered down to Pelton's Drugs on Main Street. Not long afterward, he disrobed at the Wesleyan poolside rather than in the locker room, and someone who'd previously helped him on with his shirt called and asked my mother to come and pick him up.

When my worried mother took him back to the neurologist in January 2004, he couldn't recite the months backward from May to January, even with prompting. When asked to hold up the number of fingers corresponding to the number of letters in the word "dizzy," he knew he needed to signify "five," but was totally flummoxed by how to do so with his hand. A later brain scan would discover evidence that he'd had a second, undetected stroke around this time, one that damaged the left parietal lobe of his brain, which is just beneath the crown of the head, at about the place where a yarmulke goes. The parietal lobe is a switching station, and it synthesizes images, sounds, and bodily sensations so that other parts of the brain can plan bodily movements and determine, for instance, how the hand and fingers should be configured when grasping an object.

The neurologist noted a "gradual decline" layered on top of his stroke damage, and wrote in her clinical notes that it was "conceivable that he has a mild dementia." She pondered putting him on Aricept, long the best-selling drug for dementia, which at the time cost between $150 and $200 a month. Aricept generated $2 billion in annual sales for its makers, Pfizer and Eisai Pharmaceuticals, before it lost its patent protection in 2010. Although it can be dramatically effective for a handful of patients, caregivers on the whole find it minimally effective in improving practical functioning, and some doctors prescribe it mainly to reassure relatives that "something is being done."

In retrospect, I think my father was showing signs of what I would later learn to call vascular dementia. Clots as narrow as a single human hair were lodging in tiny blood vessels in his brain, killing clusters of neurons by depriving them of oxygen. The damage affected his frontal lobes, the seat of planning and foresight directly behind the forehead, and his midbrain, which helps perform physical actions in sequence, such as knowing how to push buttons in the right order on a microwave or how to put on one's socks and shoes. The damage layered itself upon the blunderbuss destruction of at least two strokes, the mild, global brain atrophy that had occurred beforehand, and decades of normal, but cumulative, age-related cognitive decline.

*   *   *

In September 2004, three years after the stroke and two years after the insertion of the pacemaker, my mother celebrated her eightieth birthday in a rented cottage in Deer Isle, Maine. Renting the place—in fact, fussing over her birthday at all—had been my idea. But at the last minute I called with a familiar excuse: I was behind on a deadline. I sent her, instead, an eight-page homemade card, featuring Buddhist quotations, a photo-copy of the treasured family photo of my mother tucked into my father's coat in South Africa, and these lines from a painting by Paul Gauguin: "Where do we come from? Where are we going?"

The great tide that had lifted us out of our small selves had washed back. I'd become myself again—impulsive, fickle, and skittish about intimacy, especially with my mother. She went to Maine anyway, with my father and one of her closest friends. If she was angry or disappointed in me, she did not say.

After many tries, my father succeeded in writing her a short birthday letter by hand, decorated with a wavering line drawing. "You will notice I have given you the most elegant legs," he wrote in a tiny, nearly illegible script. "Your legs never let you down even though put under great pressure. Such legs are not available to every body."

My parents had a good week in Maine, and not long after they returned, my mother decided to quit Remeron on her own. I came to visit in November, got the flu, and extended my stay to a full week. Oblivious, I lay in the guest bedroom blowing my nose in my unmade bed, her calligraphy desk littered with the galleys of my finally completed magazine story.

I cooked in my mother's spotless kitchen the way I did at home—piling up mountainous salads at dinner and working my way through big plates of rice, vegetables, and chicken at lunch. My mother pursed her lips and sat down with my father, each before a translucent white plate holding half a peeled, sliced apple fanned like origami; three spears of ruffled romaine; and two or three translucent curls of sheep's milk cheese. At tea, to her annoyance, I refused her offer of toast and jam. When my father methodically wheeled out the television and turned on the evening news—one of the few chores he was still capable of doing—I declined to join her in her ritual evening glass of wine accompanied by a thimbleful of peanuts in a tiny blue and white Chinese eggcup. She asked why I deprived myself of all pleasure. I asked her to let me be. She said I was paranoid and oversensitive. The next day I borrowed a pair of socks and returned them without washing them. I withdrew to my room, nursed the tail end of my flu, and moved my return flight up by a day.

The day before I was due to leave, as we unloaded groceries from the car, she stood on her doorstep and shouted that all I thought about was "Me! Me! Me!" My diet, she said, was "rigid, excessive, and ridiculous." I could have been a teenager again, standing in the cold, tears filling my eyes. There on the doorstep, as alive as ever, were our ancient angers and griefs: my desperate need for autonomy and hers for control, our mutual inability to say, "I need you," my craving for her love, and my fury at not getting it. I ran upstairs weeping and pulled my Rollaboard out of the closet. I was nearly fifty-six, and she was eighty.

In the emotional world there is no time. Staring out the window as my Southwest flight descended once again over the Cargill salt ponds into San Francisco International Airport, I mentally ticked off my resentments: She'd told me to eat the big zucchinis and the dark chicken meat and leave her the small zucchinis and the white meat. She'd forgotten to put out a cup for me at tea. She'd mocked my father when he couldn't finish his sentences. Whenever my brothers—who barely remembered to call her on Mother's Day, while I usually sent a card or a book—hinted they needed money, she'd mail out a thousand dollars to cover a month's rent, or car insurance, or an acting workshop. But she'd insisted I pay separately for a $1.29 Burt's Bees lip balm that I'd put in her supermarket cart.

My mother called to make up. She'd just been irritated and impatient, she said, it was her besetting sin, and she was too ashamed to talk further about it. I said I wanted an apology. "Do you mean to say I habitually treat you with disrespect?" she said in surprise, and then wailed, "I have limitations!" I got off the phone and called my brothers, indulging in our cherished tradition of bashing family members behind their backs. My brother Jonathan told me to give up on the fantasy that if I played Perfect Daughter, I'd finally earn her love.

He put down the phone, found his well-thumbed copy of *The Big Book* of Alcoholics Anonymous, and read a page aloud to me:

> Acceptance is the answer to all my problems today. When I am disturbed, it is because I find some person, place, thing or situation—some fact of my life—unacceptable to me, and I can find no serenity until I accept that person, place, thing or situation as being exactly the way it is supposed to be at this moment. Nothing, absolutely nothing happens in God's world by mistake.

Over the phone, I could hear him close the book with a snap. "Your mother is a rattlesnake," he said. "She was a miserable bitch before the stroke and she's still a miserable bitch. Don't try too hard." On my next call, my brother Michael offered me empathy and called her "the cute little monster."

Lisa, one of my closest friends, who was a long-distance caregiver for an elderly, recently widowed mother and a disabled sister, advised a showdown. Some months earlier, she'd flown to New York to help her mother complete the final tax return for Lisa's deceased father. One night at 1:00 AM, when Lisa was on the phone with her husband, her mother flew into her bedroom and scolded her to put out the light and go to sleep. The next morning, Lisa sat her mother down at the breakfast table and said that at fifty-three she was old enough to choose her own bedtime, and that if this continued, she'd stop coming east to help. "Do you understand me?" she said, and would not let it go until the old woman dropped her eyes like an intimidated dog and said yes. Circumstances had changed, my friend told me. We dutiful daughters had to turn the family hierarchy upside down or perish.

The physical world was my mother's arena; I was too intimidated to confront her there. I retreated instead into the written word, and sent her a heavily revised, six-page letter of complaint, detailing every insult and every blow. "I will not be your convenient Cinderella," I wrote with a flourish, "to be praised in your hour of need and denigrated when no longer useful."

Silence.

Brian and I held a New Year's Eve party, and we all wrote down what we wanted to get rid of and what we wanted to bring into our lives, and threw the shiny papers into the blazing fireplace. One of our guests, a writer named Noelle Oxenhandler whom I then barely knew, burst into tears. Her mother, who'd been living in Provence with a lover who could no longer care for her, had dementia. Noelle, with a daughter in college and a mortgage to pay, had been forced to fly over and trick her mother into returning to the States. She set her up in a townhouse in Sonoma and was paying a full-time caregiver out of her mother's dwindling savings.

My mother and I did not speak for months. In the early spring, after teaching my annual writing workshop in Washington, DC, I took Amtrak north, stayed with an old college classmate in Larchmont, and met with editors in New York for whom I wanted to write. Then, rather than taking the Metro-North to New Haven and having my parents pick me up there, as was our custom, I went back to California. I did not want my mother to touch me with a three-thousand-mile pole.

My father kept laboring over his torturous handwritten letters to me, full of love, odd sentences, and wisdom. One letter read, "This is a bad time for you and your mother. I know you are having a 'frightful row' but that must be got over as soon as possible. You should be able to do so fairly quickly."

I did not. One day in California, I drove to the end of the box canyon I lived in, took a wooden footbridge over a stream, and climbed through a stand of second-growth redwoods and up a slope lined with blackberry bushes onto Mount Tamalpais, my sacred mountain. Up the steep railroad-tie steps to Cowboy Rock I sweated and panted, my buttocks and lungs burning, up past the county water tank and the dozen rich houses built where the Flying Y Ranch used to be. At ten in the morning, I breached a ridge and entered a vast bowl of unpopulated hills. Car sounds died away. Finches twittered in the chaparral. I followed the trail beneath a bent bay laurel, bonsaied by the winds. A madrone showed its red bones.

"Mountains," the Zen master Eihei Dogen told an assembly of Japanese monks in 1240, "are our Buddha ancestors." Inside my brain, an invisible hand turned the volume knob down. I moved deep into the sock of the valley—the only visible human. Except for a ribbon of yellow-lined asphalt below me, there was no sign of human making. Beyond the last hills lay the Pacific. Over the ridges at my back, far to the east, beyond three thousand miles of deserts and mountains, my mother was probably putting away the Manchego cheese as my father hovered around her in the kitchen. Perhaps she was shouting at him to sit down and stop crowding her. Helping her, I thought, was like reaching through barbed wire to water a rose.

*   *   *

From my earliest childhood memory, my mother was beautiful, bewildering, and dangerous. When I was four, she stopped our car on a road through a great beech woods. We were driving from Oxford to pick up my father, who was teaching in High Wycombe. It was autumn. All the leaves were golden yellow. The branches of the beeches met high above our heads, making an arched and open cathedral. The very air was yellow with the glory of the trees. My mother turned off the ignition and put the keys in her pocket. "We are going to build a house for the fairies," she said, and opened the door. We walked into the yellow woods. At a hollow place at the foot of a tree, my mother knelt. She brushed away leaves and stuck forked twigs into the ground. She balanced sticks across the clefts, making roof beams, a ridgepole, then rafters. I propped yellow leaves against the sides and roofed it in beech leaves—they were broad-bladed, like spears, and their points made a jagged line along the peak. We put moss in the front garden, and round white stones to lead the fairies to the door.

Even then she was a rebel and an agnostic, with nothing good to say about reverence. But that day she led me to something she could not give me and taught me something close to prayer. All the way back to the car, beneath the blazing beeches, I held her hand.

When had things gone wrong between us? Was it after my brother Michael was born, when I stopped serving her "tea" inside a hollowed-out bush in Oxford's University Parks? Was it the day I was five and she strolled away from me on the Woodstock Road, pushing Michael ahead in his pram, leaving me bereft on the closed, hard street to run alone, weeping, back to our locked brick row house on Thorncliffe Road, because I'd stamped my foot and argued with her about which playground to visit? Was it the evening not long after my brother Jonathan was born, when she collapsed in tears and exhaustion and my father helped her wash the boys' nappies, pulling them through the mangle with his teeth while he turned the crank with his only hand?

Was it coming to America that broke us, stripping away from our little émigré family every relative, colleague, neighbor, and friend we'd ever known? Was it building that first Techbuilt, that bare house, empty of furniture, where my father tried to finish his thesis in a dark corner of the master bedroom while my mother laid a cork floor downstairs? Was it the way my father and I treated her like an idiot because she couldn't spell? Was it her loneliness, after my father got tenure at Wesleyan and grew increasingly preoccupied with teaching, writing, and hiding out in the evenings behind his newspaper and a dark glass of bourbon and soda? Was it the day I came back from boarding school at the age of seventeen and argued with her until she slapped me in the face on the stairs of her new, bigger, better-furnished Middletown Techbuilt and I slapped her deliberately back—the only way I knew to put an end to a lifetime of her impulsive hitting and random cruelty? Was it simply that I rubbed her the wrong way because I was by nature chaotic and messy, and she was neat?

All I know is that by the time I was twelve, I hated her, and I believed she hated me—a feeling confirmed when I found a letter she was writing to my father while he was in England doing research. "Katy has been awful," it read. "But then she always was your child, anyway." I wrote my hate down in my diary, which she found and read. I hated her when she tried to teach me to sew and tore out and resewed my crooked seams until I gave up on sewing. I hated her when she grumbled, "I'm not your servant!" while cooking our dinners and cleaning our toilets and reading Betty Friedan.

After I graduated from college and spent a year working for a lawyer in Aspen, Colorado, I returned home to earn money for a couple of months before my final move to California. At one of her parties I inflated a few weeks of volunteering at the *Aspen Times* into the journalism career I dreamed of. She said sarcastically, in front of a lovely woman from San Francisco with red ringlets, "Oh! So you're a *journalist,* Katy, are you?" And yet her eyes filled with surprising tears a few weeks later as she watched me load the Rambler I'd been issued by a car transport agency, carrying a map of America, my handful of newspaper clips, and the $300 I'd earned cataloguing votes in a *My Weekly Reader* presidential poll.

When I got that Rambler stuck in a ditch in a Colorado blizzard, I did not call her for help, nor did I after I was fired from my first job in San Francisco, reading the news on an FM rock station. I didn't ask for money. I applied for unemployment and food stamps and Medicaid. I interned for an alternative weekly. I told her nothing.

I hated her on the Christmas Eve when I returned to Connecticut wearing a pair of used thirteen-button Navy pants and a new red turtleneck and green cardigan bought especially for the trip and got into my parents' car to hear my father say, "Doesn't she look nice?" and my mother say, "Too many colors." I wrote her off as a perfectionist housewife and a frustrated artist resentful of the role she was trapped in, jealous of my creative expression and childless freedom. I disdained in her everything her generation of educated, childbearing middle-class women had become and I feared becoming myself: what Adrienne Rich called "the victim in ourselves, the unfree woman, the martyr."

And all through my twenties, whenever I walked on Stinson Beach, I remembered how she longed for the long, empty sweep of the South African beaches of her childhood. When I saw a single oak rising from a cleft in the tawny flanks of Mount Tamalpais, I thought of her collecting dried wild weeds when we walked around Lake Waban in Wellesley, and how she'd cull and crop that armful of scratchy things into an arrangement of improbable, austere beauty. When I saw the Golden

Gate Bridge light up ruby in the day's last light, I'd miss her and wished she were with me.

That is how things stood between my mother and me until she and I independently discovered Buddhism. My moment of awakening came by accident when I was twenty-eight. Heading for a camping trip in the Grand Canyon, my North Beach flatmate and I decided on a whim to detour to a hot springs we'd heard about, inland from Big Sur, deep in the Ventana Wilderness. In my dusty secondhand Toyota hatchback we crawled seven miles up a winding one-lane dirt road, stopping at its highest point, Chews Ridge, to look out. All we could see were the jagged green Santa Lucia mountains, overlapped like spearheads arrayed on their sides, their knife-edges rising skyward, their bodies, enrobed with trees, flowing down into the canyons to wet their feet in Tassajara and Church Creeks, which feed the Arroyo Seco River. We got back in the car and drove the road's serpentine twists, gravity pushing us downward as I beeped at the blind turns and pumped the brakes to make sure they didn't scorch and fail. We parked in the hot dust where the road ended and walked through a massive, dark Japanese gate into a wooden settlement that looked like a cross between a medieval Buddhist monastery (which it was, in the winter) and a New Age hot springs resort (which it was, in the summer). The sign out front read, "Tassajara Zen Mountain Center: Zenshinji." It turned out that an old friend, who'd disappeared months earlier from the leftist political scene in San Francisco, was a Zen student there, and he showed us the garden, the stone *zendo,* and the "Goodwill" free closet, where you could drop off unwanted clothes and take what you needed.

I woke up at dawn in a redwood cabin, hearing running footsteps and the jangle of a handbell followed by the deliberate *Chuck! Chuck! Chuck!* of a mallet against a wooden block hung from the eaves of the meditation hall. Dressed in dark pants and a long-sleeved T-shirt, I hurried down the path in the chill, past a young man in a wide black medieval kimono limned by a white collar, as elegant as a man in a tuxedo, as he struck the final *chuckchuckchuck* roll-down on the *Han* after checking his digital watch. I put my flip-flops on a shelf, skittered down a walkway, lifted my left foot over the left threshold as I'd been shown, bowed to the gray stone Gandharan Buddha statue in the dim space, and took my seat in half-lotus on a black pebble-shaped cushion facing a white wall. I counted my deepening breaths in the safe, communal silence in a practice not so different from those that nurtured generations of my Quaker ancestors.

A handbell dinged again. My left foot was asleep. We rose. I put a flat, padded *zabuton* on the floor and, with my weight on my one good foot, made nine full bows, along with everyone else, touching my forehead to the cushion. For a religion that some adherents claimed was not a religion, it sure had a lot of ritual—more genuflecting than the Catholic Church, it seemed. Together we knelt and chanted from a translated Japanese poem that I loved but did not understand: "Yes, in darkness there is light, but don't see it as light. Yes, in light there is darkness, but don't see it as darkness." My knees hurt. We chanted some more, about filling a silver bowl with snow and hiding a heron in the moonlight. I loved the language. It pointed to something that I, a lifelong maker of phrases, couldn't put into words. "Sentient beings are numberless," we chanted. "I vow to save them." When it was over, I walked out into the clear morning light. Something nameless was within me, a pool of pure water long hidden in a covered well. I had time and I had space in a way I'd never before known. I didn't care that we chanted in languages that I didn't understand or that young men named Tommy and David and Reb had shaved their heads and put on robes and now went by Issan and Tensho and Tenshin. I wanted more.

*   *   *

When next my mother came to stay with me in San Francisco, I was living in a three-flat building I'd bought in the slums with a loan from my father, not far from the city headquarters of San Francisco Zen Center, which owned Tassajara Hot Springs. I shared it with a roommate and my brother Michael, who was then working as an electrician and also practicing Zen. Before my mother's arrival, I vacuumed out a small utility room, tucked sheets and blankets imperfectly around a single-bed mattress on the carpeted floor, and set a tiger lily in a glass jar atop a fruit crate I'd taken from the streets in Chinatown. On the bottom of the crate, I put a book for her: Zen Mind, Beginner's Mind, by the late Suzuki-Roshi, who'd founded Tassajara and my new religious home.

She was among the first off the plane and smiling—wary, pleased, and expectant. The plane had been oversold, and, thanks to her perfect blond chignon, silk scarf, and subtle jewelry, she'd been bumped to first class. On the drive home in my cluttered Toyota, she told me that sometimes the worst things in life turn out to be the best things. Breast cancer had led her to a support group run by a cancer doctor named Bernie Siegel at Yale-New Haven Hospital, and that led her to yoga and opened her mind to meditation. I was thirty then, and my mother was fifty-four. Eight years had passed since her two mastectomies. I'd seen her scarred body soon after her surgeries—she once burst into my bedroom in Middletown, naked and gesturing, "Look at me! Look at this!" The flesh over her ribs was so thin that I could see her heart pulsing. But when she was dressed, you'd never have known.

We pulled up at my building in the gentrifying and seamy Western Addition, and she made all the right noises and thanked me for the lily. Together that weekend we drove across the Golden Gate Bridge to Green Gulch Farm, a pocket in the green coastal hills of Marin County, and walked silently into Green Dragon Zen Temple, housed in a renovated bull barn. There she sat for forty minutes with her back straight and her legs folded up like everyone else's in half-lotus, facing the wall. Afterward, in a living room full of bold abstract paintings, black meditation cushions, and couches set at right angles, we listened to a shaven-headed American Zen priest whose life energy seemed to radiate palpably yet invisibly from every cell. Tears filled my mother's eyes, her hands clasping and unclasping. The priest was speaking about embracing this instant, with its joys and pains, and he picked up his teacup with a sense of the sacred that did not require a god. My mother whispered, "I've been waiting to hear this all my life."

We drove the four hours to Tassajara, down crowded Highway 101, past the lettuce fields of Salinas and the rich second homes of Carmel Valley, past a dusty trailer park on the Cachagua Road, past a scattering of houses in the settlement of Jamesburg, and finally onto the fourteen-mile dirt road over Chews Ridge, familiar to me by then. Down we went into Tassajara Canyon, trundling our bags to a small redwood cabin with a tatami-mat floor and two low futons. She was paying for me.

The Zen aesthetic accorded well with her exquisite minimalism. Outside the zendo one evening she exclaimed (loudly enough to disturb those meditating inside) over a bowl carved into a stone block, fed by water trickling from a hollowed-out bamboo stem. On a shelf in our room, a tiny glass vessel held a single bud.

We walked across an arched wooden bridge to an old stucco building whose hot springs had warmed the joints of the Esselen Indians and Victorian travelers who arrived by stagecoach, and in the 1930s, Hollywood movie stars. I slipped into the communal hot pool on the female side, joining other quiet women. My mother filled her own tub in a small private room: she was shy about her missing breasts. When I was hot enough, I stood up and made ready to head naked down the stony bank to an area of Tassajara Creek sheltered by sheets of rush matting, where other pink and naked women lay, letting the cold waters wash over them. My mother hesitated to join us, ambivalent, ashamed. "You are not doing this only for yourself," I said. "You are doing it for all the women here today who will someday get breast cancer." She took my hand and together we walked into the water.

No matter how bitterly we fought after that day—and we did—my mother was no longer only my mother to me. She was my dharma sister and my spiritual companion. The next year, when I took a leave from the *Chronicle* and worked in the Tassajara kitchen all summer, she came again to visit. She took black-and-white photographs of an elegant monk named Issan Dorsey, who had once been a meth addict, a female impersonator, and a prostitute.

My mother went home, printed and developed her photos of Issan, and took up the Japanese practice of *sumi-e,* painting the *enso,* the highest and simplest form of Zen calligraphy, making circle after bold, one-stroke circle, each a unique expression of the state of mind and body of the artist and the circumstances of its moment. From then on she would send one every Christmas to each of my brothers and to me, along with a check for three hundred dollars and a note reading "love, Ma," embellished with a heart. I gave her books like the *I Ching* and *The Tao Te Ching.*

When I was thirty-four, I wrapped myself in a white silk kimono with sleeves, lined in red silk, so deep they nearly brushed the ground. Around my waist I wound a cream raw silk obi my mother had sewn me and pinned it closed with a borrowed topaz brooch, a bowl of brimming yellow water, bought by my father decades earlier in London. My husband-to-be and I knelt on the floor of the converted bull barn as a priest named Yvonne told us to "give up your small selves and take refuge in each other."

My mother was in the front row, wearing a flowing dark red silk *aoi dai* she'd sewn herself. "I take refuge in the Buddha as the perfect teacher," I recited as she and my father watched. "I take refuge in the *sangha* as the perfect life." In one of our wedding photographs, my new husband and I run smiling through the dark carrying flowers, caught in the flash with our heads bowed, through a hail of thrown rice to the old black family Mercedes his parents had given us. Our hair is shiny, our skin unlined, our faces confident. My mother is spotlighted in the darkness in the background, and her tiny beautiful face holds the infinite sadness of a woman who knows marriage and its small deaths and quiet disappointments.

The AIDS epidemic hit, and people I loved were plunged into a medieval world of death before which medicine was powerless. Issan Dorsey, one of the Zen priests whom my mother photographed at Tassajara, founded in the Castro District of San Francisco a hospice he called Maitri, the Sanskrit word for kindness. I'd left the *Chronicle* by then, and I interviewed him for the *New Yorker*'s "Talk of the Town" section. As he patched his old summer meditation robe, he gave me a lesson on dying that went right over my head. "Half of the people in this community are going to die within the next five years," he said. "It's just our daily life. It's nothing to get out of or wish wasn't happening—it's happening.

"More and more certainly I know I'm going to die. I know people who are taking courses in the Tibetan Book of the Dead, but think it's too late for a crash course in dying. This is your preparation for dying." He put down the robe he was sewing. "Right now. Just to live your life more completely in each moment. The way I get ready for my death is by sewing these things and talking to you."

Issan died of AIDS two years later, while I was trying to avoid another kind of death, the death of my marriage, by studying the Mahayana Buddhist sutras in a monastery in southern France with the Vietnamese monk Thich Nhat Hanh. Alongside Vietnamese war-refugee nuns who knew in their bones what the words meant, I chanted every morning, "I am of the nature to grow old. There is nothing I can do to escape growing old. I am of the nature to die. There is nothing I can do to escape death." In the end, we chanted, we would lose everything and everyone precious to us. "My actions are my only true belongings," went the last lines. " I cannot escape the consequences of my actions. My actions are the ground upon which I stand."

From France I sent my mother a photograph of me smiling in a conical straw Vietnamese hat, and a watercolor I'd painted of a bursting orange flower, with this message: *Taking the first step of the day, I enter the wondrous realm of reality.* She pinned them on her bulletin board and never took them down. After I came back to America, quit my newspaper job, and separated from my husband, she listened to me cry for hours on the phone, as wrenchingly as any widow. For my next birthday, she bought me, and herself, subscriptions to *Tricycle, the Buddhist Quarterly,* and later she read the essays I wrote for it.

I was touched and surprised by her interest in Buddhism but more impressed with my own. I was the one who'd meditated at dawn in a cold stone barn for months at a time, avowed my ancient twisted karma in a black robe on the night of the full moon, studied the great master Dogen, and been given the dharma name "True Lotus" by my new teacher, Thich Nhat Hanh. I was the one who'd read the *Flower Garland Sutra* and the *Ratnakuta Sutra* and meditated on my body falling apart and becoming a rotting corpse.

Buddhism did not make my mother an easy woman, any more than it made me an easy woman. She struggled till the day she died with what 12-Steppers call character defects,

Buddhists call *samyojanas,* or internal knots, and she called her besetting sins. But after my father's stroke, it would be she, not I, who lived her Buddhism.

I rounded a ridge, and the peak of Mount Tamalpais revealed herself, rising. I remembered the Indian devotional poet Mirabai, who sang, "I worship the mountain energy night and day." I missed my mother. I wanted the pain in my heart to leave me. I wish I could tell you that my heart went out to her in her suffering or that I thought about the price she was paying for caring for my father. That I rose above myself, understood her unremitting stress, transcended being a needy and resentful daughter, and forgave her. I wish I could say that I remembered the Buddha's Second Noble Truth: that suffering is caused by wishing that things (and people) were different; and by trying with equal vehemence to stop things from changing in this evanescent world, likened by poets to a drop of dew. But thirty years of self-help groups and therapy and off-and-on Buddhist practice had done only so much for me. I still sometimes reacted like a five-year-old left in the street by a dominant and overwhelmed young mother. I was preoccupied with my own pain.

The trail switchbacked, taking me down deeper. An hour after noon, I stopped at a thick wooden memorial bench just above Muir Woods, in a grove of old-growth redwoods that the loggers left behind. There I sat, following my breath, watching my thoughts and feelings rise and fall, robed in silence and filtered brown light. The natural world restored my soul. It soothed me like a mother. I laid my burdens down before it the way I'd seen Christians at a Taizé ceremony rest their heads upon the cross.

I thought of how my mother had suffered at the hands of *her* equally critical and perfectionist mother, Agnes, who liked to say, "If there's a wrong way to do something, Val, you'll find it." I thought of Agnes's childhood tending a mother constantly felled by migraines, or "sick headaches," as they were called then. I thought of the neglected child my mother had been, with badly matched parents who didn't speak to each other for days at a time, a little girl so lonely that she fantasized being found by her parents drowned like Ophelia, who would weep over her body and finally, openly, show how much they loved her. I thought of her as a newlywed, who saw her accurate and naturalistic water-colors of exotic fish published in a landmark book, *The Sea Fishes of Southern Africa*, when she still had hopes of becoming an art-ist—until she discovered she'd accidentally become pregnant with me. How far back did it stretch, our lineage of maternal deprivation, artistic frustration, and sorrow? My female ancestors were like the orphaned lab monkeys in Harry Harlow's experi-ments, raised on cold, wire monkey-mothers, who grew up inca-pable of intuitively mothering their own.

I grew up in England after the Second World War, when the British psychoanalyst and attachment researcher John Bowlby, fascinated by the psychological effects on British chil-dren who'd been separated from their families to escape the Blitz, was studying interactions between children like me and mothers like mine. One day, two of Bowlby's successors, the researchers Mary Main and Judith Solomon, watched a little girl enter a room where her emotionally unreliable mother sat in a chair. The little girl resolved her fear and ambivalent longing by walking toward her mother backward. I had done the same. Away from her, I missed her. Next to her, I wanted to flee.

A few weeks after I came down from the mountain, I got an envelope from my mother containing some newspaper clippings she thought might interest me, and a note. She acknowledged that I'd come east without seeing them. I called her. Neither of us said I'm sorry, or I love you, or I forgive you. It was a standoff: we just went on. But in the years that followed, she would never again shout at me or criticize how I ate. She would be more tolerant. She would repeatedly tell me how much my father had loved me, and how proud of me he had been. She would, at my request, check with me before making a major medical or financial decision. She even wrote me checks so that I could hire a bookkeeper and free up my weekends to compensate for the time I spent helping her. She sent me a calligraphy reading, "Strive for imperfection."

My father never stopped writing me, and he soon sent another letter, this one containing an oblique reference to the fact that he would someday die. "All of our affection goes toward you so you must cherish it," he wrote. "Think of it often because it will sustain you." He signed it, "your Death Father."

My mother went back on Remeron, bought herself a self-help book on patience, and returned to her old comfort, Buddhist meditation. She reread a book I'd given her years earlier: *Full Catastrophe Living*, by Jon Kabat-Zinn. In it, Kabat-Zinn describes a Western form of mindfulness meditation stripped of bells, robes, and Asian religiosity. He'd introduced it to people suffering from chronic pain at a hospital in gritty Worcester, Massachusetts, and many found some relief. It was a paradox: facing and accepting the present moment, however painful, could make things feel less painful. My brother Jonathan called it accepting life on life's terms.

My mother rose alone each morning at 5:30. For the next hour and three-quarters, she was free. She slipped a Kabat-Zinn disk called *Body Scan* into the CD player I'd given her, lay down on an old padded cotton sleeping bag by the living-room window, and followed his voice, mentally sweeping her body from top to toe, releasing her diaphragm, noting each sensation, breath, mood, and thought without judgment. When the CD was finished, she did an hour's worth of yoga. Then she went upstairs, got my father up, and began yet another day—a day whose stresses increased with each stage of my father's decline. She wrote in her journal that she found herself more patient, responding rather than reacting. She felt she could face whatever came her way.

For Christmas 2005, a little more than a year after our blowup, I came home. It was four years since the stroke, and my father was now eighty-two: quieter, more easily fatigued and confused, and more unsteady on his feet. He was still exercising at the pool, but Toni now drove him there. The second upstairs bathroom had been renovated since my last visit; my mother brought in a construction crew and replaced the tub with a walk-in handicapped shower.

I took my father with me one evening to steal a frond of dry bamboo from the Japanese garden behind Wesleyan's Asian Arts Center—the kind of petty larceny that my mother and I loved to indulge in, and that had once sent him into paroxysms of embarrassment. We brought it home in the darkness, and my father hung up his own coat—my mother had finally moved the hook down to where he could reach it. We strung the bamboo stalk with shiny Christmas globes and tiny lights.

My mother roasted a duck for Christmas dinner, and we invited over one of my parents' friends, a dying architect named T.J., who'd designed the vestibule added on to my parents' house. His wife died a month earlier of breast cancer at home under hospice care. T.J. had congestive heart failure, and the West African woman caring for him drove his station wagon through our backyard, across a snowy slope in the darkness, to get him as close as possible to my parents' sliding glass back door. My mother and I stood on either side of him as a light snow fell, and we helped him in.

Even though Brian and I usually gave holiday dinners for his sons and his old friends, Christmas had not meant much to me for a long time. When I was in my twenties and broke, my parents never offered to pay for my flight east. When I worked for the newspaper, especially after my divorce, I often worked the holiday for the time-and-a-half overtime pay. But as the four of us sat in our tippy bentwood chairs around the long oak table my mother had bleached and refinished—my father and T.J. so quiet, my mother and I so talkative—I remembered times of grace.

On our last Christmas Eve in Oxford, a young boy in a cap had come to our door in the snowy twilight, opened his hymnal, and started singing. I stood behind the leaded glass listening as my mother whispered, *Wait, don't open the door yet, listen.* I still remember him there, the snow falling in the lamplight on his cap and his hymnal, his clear, pure voice singing "Silent Night," and when I opened the door, the sudden stop of his singing. My mother handed me a silver shilling to give him; he took it, closed his book, thanked me, and was gone.

I remembered another Christmas Eve, my third in America, the year I turned eleven. It was 1960, John Kennedy had recently been elected president, and we'd put up our first Christmas tree in the new Techbuilt overlooking the lake on the outskirts of Wellesley. I'd spent the day at the house of my best friend, Janet, whose mother's alcoholism was well advanced. There were lots of grown-ups there that day, drinking and smoking and playing guitar in the kitchen. Janet cooked us a lunch of canned SpaghettiOs, and the adults forgot about us. It began to snow, and by nightfall the highway that ran the three miles from Janet's house to my own was closed.

By then, my closeness to my father was long gone—lost to our nightly dinner-table arguments and his terrified preoccupation with his own work. I thought I would spend the night with Janet's family, and nobody would much care. Then my father called to say he would walk halfway to meet me. It was a long cold way to go alone, but as I walked through the falling snow, from streetlamp to streetlamp along the soft, silent highway, I was not afraid. It was a beautiful night, and the snow, caught in the streetlamps, sparkled as it whirled and fell. The memory was precious to me, a reminder of how much my father loved me. He was there to meet me halfway, and not angry, and together we walked home.

I put down my napkin, and my mother helped my father unloop his. We helped T.J. back to his car, said good-bye to him for what turned out to be the last time, and blew the candles out.

Under the bamboo branch that my mother and I had hung with baubles, I found, the next morning, a beautifully wrapped present. It was a paperback book called *Best Buddhist Writing 2005*. On the frontispiece, my mother had written out part of verse 41 of the *Tao Te Ching* that I'd given her years before:

Dearest Katy
The path into the light seems dark,
The path forward seems to go back,
The direct path seems long,
True power seems weak . . .
True clarity seems obscure . . .
The Tao is nowhere to be found,
Yet it nourishes and completes all things.

Love, Ma.

CHAPTER 9

BROKE-DOWN PALACE

Full fathom five thy father lies;
Of his bones are coral made;
Those are pearls that were his eyes:
Nothing of him that doth fade
But doth suffer a sea-change
Into something rich and strange.

—ARIEL, IN *The Tempest*, WILLIAM SHAKESPEARE

From the perspective of an electron microscope, the young healthy brain is like a net hung with jewels, a complex web of branching and interconnected nerve cells chattering to one another through long filaments, playing enormous games of gossip, sucking up and spitting out neurochemicals, and passing on messages to their neighbors via tiny charges of electricity. From a greater distance, the brain could be envisioned as an enormous city, bigger than Jakarta, composed of clusters of semi-independent neighborhoods, eighty-six billion neurons strong, connected via electrochemical freeways, alleys, dirt paths, donkey routes, thoroughfares, and side streets. When one freeway in the brain collapses, messages often get through by other pathways. When a neighborhood specializing, say, in finding words is obliterated by a stroke, cells in other neighborhoods try to pick up part of the work, with varying degrees of success. The healthy brain, like the healthy young heart and body, is full of programmed redundancies, work-arounds, and backup routes. Neurologists call this resilience "cognitive reserve."

But at the astonishingly early age of twenty-two, some parts of the neural city begin to decay, even as others—such as those involved in bridling impulsivity, thinking through decisions, regulating emotion, and gaining mastery over complex crafts such as journalism, teaching, or cabinetmaking—continue to elaborate. Each year, scores on standardized tests of short-term memory, reasoning, reaction time, dexterity, rapid generation of new ideas, and speed of learning fall by up to 1 percent. Great breakthroughs in fields such as chemistry, mathematics, and physics—as in athletics—are usually the work of people in their late twenties and early thirties. Our brains shrink. Dendritic spines, the knobby lumps on individual brain cells that act as contact points between neurons, grow sparse and stubby, like a tree limb that has been harshly pruned. Synapses fail, and associated neural pathways fall into disuse. Arteries thicken, reducing blood flow. Myelin, the fatty white protective sheath that surrounds filamental brain cells like insulation, grows as porous and leaky as an old hose, slowing the speed at which messages move from one cell to another. Even as we grow more deliberate, emotionally skilled, and patient, we understand what people say to us more slowly, and our thinking grows less sharp.

In our fifties, levels of hormones fall noticeably, including several, such as estrogen, androgen, and dopamine, that enhance memory, mood, and focus. We forget names. We fumble more with tweezers. We get distracted when too many people talk at once. For a long time, minor losses of brainpower remain invisible to us and our friends and perceptible only on standardized tests. Our brains' multiple work-arounds keep working. The cunning, wisdom, and accumulated knowledge of middle age triumph over ignorant and impulsive youth.

The declines accelerate after age sixty. Proteins, badly copied, fold into odd shapes inside cells and clog things up. Tangles of dead cellular material—a defining biological hallmark of Alzheimer's disease but occurring in smaller quantities in the brains of the sharp-minded as well—block neural highways like uncollected garbage. Inflammation takes a toll. Shrinkage occurs in the hippocampus, a seahorse-shaped brain region deep in the skull that shuttles memories from short-term to long-term brain storage. We take longer to learn languages and to operate new electronic devices.

The pauses that follow the search for a name grow longer. We drive more slowly to compensate for our slower reaction times. We joke about "senior moments." Minor cellular damage accumulates, and neural work-arounds grow scarcer. Depending on how broadly the damage is defined, 10 to 30 percent of people over sixty-five exhibit what neurologists call "mild cognitive impairment," an umbrella term for mental decline that is bad enough to be worrisome but not yet severely disabling. It includes forgetting important appointments and conversations, having difficulty making decisions, misplacing keys and reading glasses, and paying the same bills twice. We adapt. We keep stricter appointment books and follow rigid, easy-to-remember schedules, becoming set in our ways. Yet we remain, we think, fundamentally ourselves.

What happened to my father between 2005 and 2008—the final three years of his life, the years his doctors thought he would not have lived to see without his pacemaker—was worse than that.

To the end of his days, he never wandered away from home, or had to be confined or tied up, or forgot my face or my name, or drooled, or thought he saw the faces of the dead, or dandled a baby doll in his arms, or insisted it was time he got dressed and off to work. He never became blissfully unaware of his decline. He still remembered the pattern of Hartford's twisting streets and freeway on-ramps, and acted as navigator when Toni took him there to the eye doctor. He had islets of competence. He remained, to the end, my dear father Jeff.

But there came a time when the losses mounted beyond what a human being could bear to watch or to endure. Or should be forced to by an act of medicine.

His brain cells did not simply lose their dendritic spines, as occurs in ordinary aging. They died in large enough numbers to obliterate neural pathways connecting areas of the brain that took in what he saw and sensed with those designed to form plans to do something about it. Dr. Fales, my father's internist, came to think of those years as "Jeff's Ordeal." Exactly what he had feared came to pass. "My heart went out to what your parents went through," he said to me years later. "Particularly your mother, because she experienced watching him, being his partner of so many years." The age-related degeneration that had earlier slowed my father's heart and shrunk his brain moved on to attack his eyes, lungs, bladder, and bowels. He was collapsing slowly, like an ancient, shored-up house.

In June 2005, my father complained of double vision and was diagnosed with wet macular degeneration in his right eye, a rogue overgrowth of blood vessels in the retina that leads to blindness. It is caused by accumulating DNA glitches that allow the replication of cells that shouldn't replicate, a process that occurs throughout the aging body, leading to funny growths as harmless as skin tags and as deadly as cancer. The extra blood vessels formed a black spot at the center of my father's field of vision. "There is not much that one can do about it; one just suffers from it with age," he wrote to me philosophically. The localized blindness layered itself upon a sight already globally dimmed by time; proteins in the crystalline lenses of our eyes grow stiff and yellowed with age, like a dirty window. The eye of even a healthy sixty-year-old lets in one third as much light as the eye of someone of twenty.

Thus my father entered the second-to-last stage of the long chess match with death that we play with such absorption and lose with such surprise. Things that should be supple, such as arteries, grow stiff, and things that should be strong, such as bones, grow porous. Some cells die and aren't replaced. Cartilage and collagen thin. Calcium is pulled from bones and dumped into arteries. According to author-surgeon Atul Gawande, the aorta and other major blood vessels in the elderly "often feel crunchy under your fingers" during heart surgery. Bone spurs sprout on femurs and knee joints like knobs of coral. Some cells undergo destructive metabolic processes called "browning," analogous to rusting or slow cooking. Muscles wither with disuse. The ends of our cellular DNA lose a few last notes of code with every replication, increasing the likelihood of cancerous mutations. The longer we live, the more our brains and bodies are pummeled by what Shakespeare called "the thousand natural shocks the flesh is heir to."

What we call aging is the cumulative effect of more than seven thousand separate degenerative bodily processes, each shaped by our genes, habits, and environment. Sentinel cells in the bloodstream devour fewer invading microbes and increase the chances of succumbing to the flu, bronchitis, a urinary tract infection, or pneumonia. Even our ability to regulate our body temperature weakens. Our optimistic, science-worshipping culture wants to medicalize aging and make it nothing more than a collection of specific diseases that medicine can prevent or fix, one item at a time. But no matter what deal we make with the devil, nature outwits us. Dying can be postponed, but aging cannot be cured. Although brilliant minds hunt for a longevity gene, and life-extension Web sites hawk acai berries and selenium, science so far has not found a way around the eternal truth that propelled the Buddha into a lifetime of meditation and that I blithely recited in monasteries in my forties: *there is no way to escape growing old.*

*   *   *

To slow, stop, or hopefully even reverse his descending blindness, Toni drove my father once a month to an ophthalmologist in Hartford who injected his right eyeball with an expensive drug called Macugen (pegaptanib), made jointly by Pfizer and a smaller company called Eyetech Pharmaceuticals. It wasn't terribly effective. Not long afterward, the ophthalmologist tried out another drug, Avastin (bevacizumab), made by a Bay Area biotech company, Genentech.

Licensed as a chemotherapy for several cancers, Avastin retards the growth of blood vessels, such as those that feed tumors. It was sold in bulk in big, sealed plastic bags. It cost only fifty dollars per injection when divided up by specialized "compounding pharmacies" into microdoses for the eye. At a professional conference, doctors who'd tried it told my father's ophthalmologist that it was much more effective than Macugen, and so he switched. Then Genentech released a much more expensive drug, Lucentis (ranibizumab), specifically designed, approved, and promoted for macular degeneration. Many doctors continued to use the cheaper Avastin "off-label" (that is, for a purpose not licensed by the Food and Drug Administration) rather than switching to Lucentis (which later studies proved no more effective than Avastin), especially for their poorer and more poorly insured clients. But my father had Medicare and good supplementary insurance, and Lucentis was the officially approved treatment, so my father's doctor went with Lucentis.

Each Lucentis dose cost Medicare about $1,560 and my father's supplemental insurance about $389—roughly the cost of a year of my father's speech therapy. The total charge per forty-five-minute office visit averaged $2,127, of which about $178 went directly to the ophthalmologist for giving the shot. In 2005 and 2006 alone, fourteen months' worth of Lucentis injections cost Medicare $18,723 and my father's supplemental insurance $4,678, for a total of close to $25,000—money that would probably not have been spent had my father died a timely natural death. Medicare allows doctors to mark up the cost of drugs they use by roughly 6 percent, so the ophthalmologist, who did not respond to my requests for billing information, may have earned an additional $3 each time he used Avastin and up to $120 extra when he used Lucentis.

The treatments did not help. According to the doctor's records, my father's sight got dramatically worse. Month after month, Toni said, he couldn't make out a single letter on the eye chart. She thought the visits did more for the bottom lines of the doctor and the drug companies than they did for my Dad.

By then, Toni and my mother were regularly ferrying my father to a cavalcade of doctors. All ran tests, wrote reports, kept dutiful records, billed Medicare, tracked my father's decline, and did little to coordinate with one another. A technician from Middlesex Cardiology Services checked the pacemaker once every three months by a remote phone hookup, and twice every year, my mother and father went in for an office visit with Dr. Rogan to make sure his heart and his pacemaker were still functioning properly.

My father wrote me fewer letters. When I asked to speak to him on the phone, he shouted out testily, "What for?" and fumbled with the receiver. He could no longer place a phone call on his own. For a while I shouted back, "I love you," and then I gave up.

The functioning of the brain is influenced by shifting tides of neurochemicals, and my father's mind grew temporarily sharper—this is what's so confusing about dementia—when he was in a buoyant mood. In the spring of 2006, I published a freelance article in the science section of the *New York Times*— my first for the paper—and got a short, excited handwritten note from him. "I am writing to you in a great hurry to catch you before you land here," he wrote. "We are delighted with your *Times* article about sibling violence. Yesterday I spent the whole day thinking of it.

"The idea is first-class—the taking of an ordinary idea and seeing what can be done with it," he went on. "I was intrigued at your using the example of Cain killing Abel. It is a marvelous example of brothers going at each other."

He even ventured the sort of pedantic editing that had demoralized me when I was younger. He asked for a definition of "siblicide," pointed out what he called "mixed-up language" in a sentence he didn't like, and said he was baffled by my unexplained reference to Craigslist. "Is it some kind of list defined and classified on some basis and mixed up with a Web site? These are things to look out for." My heart lifted. I had, for a moment, my old father back. Not bad, I thought, for a stroke-ridden man of eighty-three who'd rarely used the Internet. I was as proud of him as he was of me.

When I had breakfast with him in Middletown two weeks later, however, the neurological weather had changed. He slumped more and spoke less. He no longer helped my mother set the table. Every now and again, his left eye would go dull and wander, as though a cloud was passing through his brain, then he'd refocus and pick up his spoon again. He needed help looping his blue-checked napkin over his head on its stretchy black ribbon, and he didn't fold it and pat it and put it away ritually after breakfast anymore, leaving it crumpled instead for my mother to put away. He followed her from room to room and hovered about her in the kitchen, a phenomenon I later learned was called "shadowing."

The pacemaker kept on ticking.

*   *   *

Leaving my father behind with Toni, I took my reluctant mother (who hated the word "dementia" almost as vehemently as she hated thinking about the future) to see a counselor at the closest office of the Alzheimer's Association, near New Haven. The counselor showed us a set of charts of declining mental function. They reminded me of stock market trajectories in a series of bad years, squiggling ever downward, with the stroke victims falling abruptly down staircases after each "cardiovascular event" and the Alzheimer's sufferers trundling more gently down sloping foothills. My father seemed to be failing in both ways at once: his plateaus were sometimes followed by sudden drops and sometimes by gentle declines. I looked at the charts and wondered: Should I keep nagging my mother to extend Toni's hours or even, God help us, to put him in an adult day care program? Did he have Alzheimer's disease as well?

Given how much is unknown about the more than fifty causes and risk factors of mental decline and dementia—among them obesity, depression, alcoholism, cardiac surgery, chemotherapy, diabetes, mutated cells, a high-fat diet, genetics, a sedentary life, social isolation, depression, and just plain old age—my last question was probably irrelevant. Like cancer, "dementia" remains a catchall label rather than a diagnosis, sheltering a miscellany of poorly understood diseases, maladies, and age-related deficits under one tattered umbrella. It is to the twenty-first century what tuberculosis was to the nineteenth century and AIDS to the twentieth: a widespread, dreaded, fatal, and incurable pariah condition, filled with shame.

On the advice of the Alzheimer's counselor, I went to Staples and bought my parents two small whiteboards, one to tack on the door of the upstairs study, and another for the kitchen. My plan was to have my mother post their daily schedule there, thus reducing the number of times my father asked her over and over about their plans. She took the one downstairs for her grocery lists, and put the other one in an upstairs closet.

Half a billion federal dollars are spent each year on Alzheimer's research, but an estimated 20 to 40 percent of dementias are not caused by classic Alzheimer's and will not be fixed even if the elusive cure (or cures) for that enigmatic malady (or maladies) is ever found. (All dementias not otherwise classified are now lumped into the Alzheimer's diagnosis.) "Dementia" is a practical term: it means simply that brain deterioration has reached a tipping point and the sufferer can no longer function safely without help. Much about it is not well understood. And while hip joints can be replaced, and the heart's clogged tubes and failing pumps can be reamed out and reinforced with artificial parts, the aging brain is too complex, gelatinous, and delicate to fix like a machine. Neurons die and don't come back. Despite repeated hopeful scientific announcements of breakthrough drugs, new diagnostic tests, and genetic discoveries, there remains no pacemaker for the brain, no penicillin, and no Botox.

Dementias can be avoided more easily than cured. A quick Internet search suggested that if I wanted to escape my father's fate, I should become a happy, hardy vegan who weighed less than average, had normal blood pressure, drank coffee or tea, was literate, well-off, and well-educated, kept up with friends and interesting hobbies, went to church, gave to others but not too much, took ibuprofen and estrogen, drank red wine but not too much, exercised hard, avoided salt, sugar, saturated fat, and white flour, had a lucky gene associated with longevity without dementia, and had been capable in my twenties of writing a complex and coherent life narrative.

My father had exercised regularly and eaten healthfully. He had normal blood pressure and had been rangy, literate, well-off, and well-educated. He kept up with his friends and interesting hobbies, gave to others but not too much, drank tea and coffee, and had certainly been capable, in his twenties, of writing a complex and coherent life narrative.

Maybe it would be better to die before dementia struck.

The Alzheimer's Association, in service of one of its primary missions, which is to promote expanded funding for research, has long sought to differentiate Alzheimer's from "normal aging." (Research dollars don't go to conditions but to diseases, which by definition have potential cures.) But although a few rare variants strike early, the fact remains that longevity is the biggest risk factor for cognitive decline and for most dementias, including Alzheimer's. The damage hits home hard after eighty: only 9 percent of those seventy and over have dementia, while among those eighty and over, at least one-third do. For those who reach ninety, the chances of leaving this world lucid become little better than a coin toss: more than 41 percent of those ninety and over have dementia, at least another 10 to 15 percent have mild cognitive impairment, and only one in two hundred has no trace of cognitive decline. Each medical advance that fixes the body without helping the mind increases widespread survival into extreme old age and fuels the dementia epidemic.

From there the ripples spread. The democratization of longevity, which amplified the dementia epidemic, is also responsible for the caregiving crisis. Wealth, traditionally transferred from one generation to the next, now flows instead into the treasuries of assisted-living chains, long-term insurance providers, home-care companies, and nursing homes. (Medicare, with rare time-limited exceptions, does not cover long-term skilled nursing care.)

In the last five years of their lives, a quarter of the elderly now spend all of their savings, including the value of their homes, on caregiving and other out-of-pocket medical expenses. Forty-three percent lose everything except their homes. Those with dementia, of course, pay the most. This represents a stunning evaporation of the capital transfers that traditionally helped families become upwardly mobile or maintain their shaky perches in a beleaguered middle class. Gone is the inherited family homestead, the $5,000 bequest for a grandchild's car or first year at a community college, the $25,000 loan or gift toward a house down payment, or, in wealthier families, $100,000 toward starting a business, paying off a mortgage, or covering tuition for grandchildren's college or graduate school.

"We are now in a post-stroke mode and have to look after ourselves," my father wrote to me elegiacally in the late spring of 2006:

> Before we depended on old Jeff but now Val is strictly in command. If you look at this house and garden it really is beautiful. Val has gone to enormous trouble and I am afraid she has done it all. But a few things I have done. In particular, I have taken on the sorting of sand and gravel. It really was a terrible mess and I set myself the task of sorting it out. If you walked along the deck you would see what it is that I am talking about. So my dear, you are the recipient of a tortured piece, by a man who tries to sort things out on the ground.

What did it feel like, I wonder, to peer out at the world through the shifting keyholes of that generous soul and educated mind, with a black spot in his field of vision and his ears stopped with hearing aids that he could no longer put in without help? What was it like to have holes appear and disappear in memory like film jammed in a projector and melting? What was it like, after a life-time of overcoming hardship and adapting to limitation without complaint, not to recognize a road he'd walked for forty years or to watch his hand write the word "rhetoric" over and over?

And yet, my father in ruin was in some ways more beautiful to me than my father intact. I could see more clearly the outlines of his soul. He let go, by necessity, of what Shakespeare called "the bubble reputation" and Ecclesiastes called vanity and vexation of soul. He would never finish his book or his memoir, redeem his delinquent boyhood, make his dead father proud, or eclipse his better-known, long-resented, and now thoroughly dead older brother Guy, the poet. My father could no longer strive and do. He could only love and be loved. The race was run.

"When a fine old carpet is eaten by mice, the colors and patterns of what's left behind do not change," wrote my neighbor and friend, the poet Jane Hirshfield, after she visited an old friend suffering from Alzheimer's disease in a nursing home. And so it was with my father. His mind did not melt evenly into undistinguishable lumps, like a dissolving sand castle. It was ravaged selectively, like Tintern Abbey, the Cistercian monastery in northern Wales suppressed in 1531 by King Henry VIII in his split with the Church of Rome. Tintern was turned over to a nobleman, its stained-glass windows smashed, its roof tiles scavenged for their lead, its church bells melted, its floor tiles taken up and relaid in village houses. Holy artifacts were sold to passing tourists. Religious statues turned up in nearby gardens. At least one interior wall was dismantled to build a pigsty.

I've seen photographs of the remains that inspired Wordsworth: a Gothic skeleton, soaring and roofless, in a green hilly landscape. Grass grows in the transept. The vanished roof lets in light. The delicate stone tracery of its slim, arched quatrefoil windows opens onto green pastures where black-and-white cows graze. Its shape is beautiful, formal, and mysterious. After he developed dementia, my father was no longer useful to anybody. But in the shelter of his broken walls, my mother learned to balance her checkbook, and my heart melted and opened. Never would I wish upon my father the misery of his final years. But he was sacred in his ruin, and I took from it the shards that still sustain me.

CHAPTER 10

WHITE WATER

On June 4, 2006, my mother opened her journal after a three-year hiatus. "Today, Sunday, a very disturbing development in Jeff's behavior," she wrote:

> He is repeating and repeating cleaning his teeth. It all started on Friday when we bought a new water pick. Any new procedure throws him, but today he was close to crazy in the afternoon—kept going upstairs to the bathroom and cleaning his teeth. I got him to do some cutting of vinca minor in the front as he has done in the past. He took a long time but managed to do a little. But as soon as he got inside he started for the bathroom and began the tooth cleaning. After supper he could not wait to go upstairs again to clean his teeth.

My father's neurologist had earlier told us that this kind of repetitive behavior—previously confined to getting stuck like a broken record on a repeated phrase, or checking and rechecking the calendar—is called *perseveration*. It is commonplace among the autistic and the otherwise brain-damaged. On nuclear imaging tests, it correlates with decreased blood flow to the outer layer of two folded outer bulges of brain behind the forehead called the frontal lobes, especially an area called the dorsal prefrontal cortex, where neurons act as traffic cops, switching attention from one word or action to something new. Damage to the frontal lobes may be the most tragic of all mental losses, because the lobes carry out many functions vital to the empowered adult self: the ability to act morally, to make decisions, to think through the consequences of actions, to problem solve, and to make a plan and carry it through.

"Perseverence, perseverence, perseverence!!!!" my mother continued in her journal, misspelling the word in her agony:

> Oh God now it's like he is totally insane, and I am not sure of what to do next. I will wait for the morning and hope that he has slept it off. I am anxious and upset and do not want to have a sleepless night because of it. I will do my stress reduction tape and hope it helps me, but I feel my blood pressure must be sky high as a result of frustration with Jeff. He just won't listen but goes on with his OBSESSION. Is this Alzheimer's? It certainly is dementia.
>
> I feel my life is in ruins. This is horrible and I have lasted for five years. Sometimes I wish he would die and set me free.

That night she played the relaxation tape I'd sent her, returned to her morning meditation the next day, and wrote in the journal again in a calmer mood. She was attempting to control her impatience and anger, and my father, she wrote, was much better for it. She decided to accept what her life, and her husband, had become. "I now acknowledge fully that the Jeff I married and lived with for sixty years is no longer the same person," she wrote. "Jeff is querulous, anxious, and resentful and expects me to know everything and attend, attend, to his needs. I try to respond in a neutral way and simply get on with what I want to do."

Other wives let go by taking off their wedding rings. One found relief by thinking of her demented husband as a new member of the family, an entirely different person from the man she'd married. A woman of the Anishinabe tribe in northern Minnesota held a funeral for her demented mother while she was still living. "We lost the mother that we once knew . . . she is the child now and I am the mother," she told the social psychologist Pauline Boss, who coined the term "ambiguous loss" to describe what these women were experiencing.

My mother did not tell me about that weekend. Only after her death, when I read her whole journal, would I understand how much she'd tried to shield her children from the misery engulfing her and my father. She conducted her sacrament of relinquishment alone.

She told me only that she was reading *Elegy for Iris,* John Bayley's obituary for his then-still-living wife, the brilliant English novelist Iris Murdoch, tracking her descent into dementia. On the phone with me, my mother repeated the book's most famous phrase, from an unnamed woman who told Bayley that life with her demented husband was "like being chained to a corpse." She reread Edith Hamilton's books about the Greeks, and sent me a quote from Aeschylus: "And even in our sleep, pain that cannot forget falls drop by drop upon the heart, and in our own despite, against our will, comes wisdom to us by the awful grace of God."

*   *   *

On June 9, 2006, my mother found my father crumpled in the driveway, moaning, unable to get himself up, one eye covered in blood. She called 911. She'd gone down to the street with him to bring in the garbage cans, and afterward she'd told him to walk to the house alone while she visited a next-door neighbor. It was far from the first time he'd fallen, but it was the worst. A CAT scan at Middlesex Hospital showed cracked bones in his right eye socket, plus evidence of a previously undetected stroke on the left side of his brain near the back of the head that had probably occurred in 2003. There were signs of a separate brain bleed behind the cracked bones near his right temple. It wasn't clear whether he'd had a brain hemorrhage and fallen, or fallen and had a brain hemorrhage. Doctors sent him by ambulance to Yale–New Haven Hospital, an hour away, to be evaluated for brain surgery.

The hospital, in the poor city of New Haven, was a training ground for Yale Medical School's interns and residents. Its emergency room, like those of most urban hospitals, was a clinic of last resort for the uninsured poor. My mother stayed up much of the night in a hallway outside the crowded ER, while my father lay next to her on a gurney, tossing and muttering. She told me he waited more than a day for a bed.

Yale–New Haven was ranked among the top 3 percent of U.S. hospitals in ten advanced specialties that year, including neurosurgery, according to *U.S. News & World Report*. Sending him there might have been a mistake. There is no necessary relationship between the size and sophistication of a hospital and the quality of its nursing care, and when you are frail, the simplest touch from a good nurse can matter more than a high-tech specialty. I later discovered, in ratings assembled by a respected consumer magazine from government data, that Middletown's little Middlesex Memorial Hospital was rated the safest of the twenty hospitals in Connecticut. Yale–New Haven ran fourth-to-last, with high rates of hospital-acquired infections and readmissions not long after discharge and low scores on doctors' and nurses' communications with patients about important things such as how to take care of sutures and what pills to take once they were released.

After my mother left to get some sleep, orderlies failed to notice that my father had only one arm and did not help him to eat or drink. Neither she nor I knew then that many hospitals have become, in the words of one bereaved-son-turned-investigative-journalist, places that provide "bodily repair services under the direction of independent physician-scientists," where over-stretched nurses provide monitoring but very little old-fashioned nursing care. My father grew hungry, thirsty, and disoriented, lashing out at things that weren't there. He was suffering from what doctors call "hospital delirium," a state of temporary hallucination, confusion, and disorientation that affects about one-third of hospital patients over seventy. It can be triggered by not having one's hearing aids or eyeglasses, by medication errors or anesthesia, and by a toxic hospital environment that somehow passes for normal: noise as loud and constant as a highly trafficked street; being wakened in the middle of the night for blood pressure readings that could be done in daylight; harried aides; lack of needed help to drink water or eat the terrible food; an absence of reassuring human touch; not being spoken to by name; and windowless, eternally lighted rooms that, like casinos, eliminate all sense of day and night.

On top of this, hospitals today usually lack the three healing conditions that the Victorian-era nursing reformer Florence Nightingale considered essential: quiet, rest, and fresh air. Of those who suffer hospital delirium, 35 to 40 percent die within a year.

My mother called me, weeping. She was exhausted. The hospital was neglecting him. She was afraid to drive alone to New Haven. She didn't know what to do. She needed a driver. She needed a medical advocate. She needed me.

A Korean folk saying holds that after three years of caregiving, filial devotion disappears. I was lying on the couch worn-out when I got her call, looking up at the skylight. It had been five years of back-and-forth flights, three of them in the previous eight months. Brian and I were packing for a nonrefundable week at a rented cabin in the mountains. I did not know how many more years my father would last, and after that—what then? My mother's mother lived to be ninety-two. My mother might well live as long, which meant I'd be taking care of her when I was seventy. And after that—how many years would it be before Brian, whom I'd so far resisted marrying for reasons I didn't fully understand, needed my care? Who would be left in the end to care for me? And why did most of the burden fall on women? I called my brothers. It was their turn, I said. After completing a weeklong acting workshop that he'd already paid for, my brother Michael flew out. It was only his second visit home since my father's stroke.

Much to my relief, the doctors at Yale–New Haven decided not to operate—a wise "less is more" decision for which the hospital paid a financial price. Out of $22,034 in services billed, Medicare reimbursed the hospital only $6,668 under its lump-sum system—a figure that would have been far higher, of course, if doctors had subjected my father to brain surgery. All in all, the six-day hospitalization cost Medicare about $16,891, including $8,723 for emergency, diagnostic, and doctors' services at Middlesex Memorial the first day and $1,500 for separately-billed doctors' services at Yale–New Haven.

My mother insisted on bringing my father home as soon as she could. He never returned to his previous "normal." One morning, while sitting on the couch, he asked my brother Michael why the room was filling up with leaves. In hindsight, he'd have been better off if my mother had not called 911 after his fall but just washed the blood off his face and put him to bed.

*   *   *

If my parents' seventies were golden years, their eighties were years of lead. For the first two years after his stroke—2002 and 2003—my father and mother organized their lives around their hope of his getting better, her determination to help him, and his fierce motivation to regain the ability to write and speak. When hope of true recovery ended, they marched on, my mother growing ever more lonely and exhausted, and my father accepting a constricted life of limited but real pleasures. The fourth and fifth poststroke years—2005 and 2006—took from them even the most limited pleasures. My father's sight dimmed so much that he could no longer read the *New York Times*. His balance became so unsteady that my mother no longer let him walk on his own and held him up by his belt when he walked up or down stairs. He became bowel and bladder incontinent, and that meant the end of his water walking at the Wesleyan pool and his lunches out twice a month with his old colleague Richard Adelstein. His brain became so damaged that he could not form a plan to get to the bathroom on time when he needed to, but not damaged enough to keep him from being ashamed and remorseful when Toni or my mother had to wipe the shit from his bottom.

His life went on, thanks perhaps to his pacemaker, and he could do nothing about it but endure. The tipping point had come. Death would have been a blessing, and living was a curse. As he put it to my mother one day, in his classic understated style, "Unfortunately, I come from long-lived people." As Toni remembered it, "He was confined to the house, and that was horrible. He would sit in a chair with a book and just sit there. There was nothing left for him. The only time I saw him happy was when you visited. When you were around, he was *on the page*. He adored you: you were Daddy's little girl. Otherwise, it was take a nap, take a nap, there was nothing else left. He liked to eat, and that was it."

*   *   *

In California, I woke up some mornings in a fury. Why had his doctors not let nature take its course? If the pacemaker had never been implanted, I thought, my father might well have been out of his misery, and so would my mother and I be. I understood very little about the device then, and I thought that the only way to disable it was to subject my father to a second surgery—a path that seemed unthinkably cruel, dangerously close to euthanasia, and, practically speaking, impossible. I did not curse the mysterious ways of God, in whom I did not believe, for keeping my father alive. I cursed the machinery of man for disrupting the natural order, which over millions of years of evolution had designed our hearts and brains to fail at pretty much the same time. Where was Dr. Rogan now, I wondered, to see what my father's bonus years had brought? Would he come over to my parents' house on Pine Street and look after my father for a single day?

When I called my brother Jonathan and vented, he joked darkly about putting a pillow over my father's head. I told him about Temple Lee Stuart, a woman who lived one town away from me in Sausalito. She'd pled guilty to manslaughter and was sentenced to six years in prison for smothering her eighty-eight-year-old mother with a pillow in her nursing home bed. The daughter called it a mercy killing, and maintained that her mother had repeatedly said she wanted to die. Temple had been the only one of her mother's children who regularly visited the old lady. Temple had confessed to a brother who lived out of town and was arrested after he turned her in.

On New Year's Eve at the close of 2006, the worst, most hopeless year so far of my father's long life, I wrote out a prayer in my despair and put it into my "God Box"—a coffee can onto which I'd glued National Geographic shots of canyons, African rock paintings, and other images of the sacred that I craved, despite my lack of conventional religious belief. A friend in a 12-step program had recommended it as a technique for letting go of what could not be fixed. "Please take care of my mother," I wrote. "Lead her to respite. Help me let go of trying to control her and solve all of her problems. Help me flourish creatively and personally whether she is happy or not. Please help her let go, and let Jeff die."

IV

REBELLION

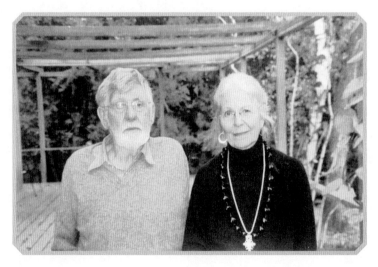

Jeffrey and Valerie Butler, Pine Street, Middletown, Connecticut, 2006.

CHAPTER 11

THE
SORCERER'S APPRENTICE

I n January 2007, five months after my father's disastrous stay
at Yale–New Haven Hospital, I interviewed a woman named
Katrina Bramstedt who worked for the Cleveland Clinic. I
did not immediately understand how her work applied to my
family's dilemmas, but soon enough I would. I was looking for
science stories to write, and she was a hospital bioethicist, a
member of a relatively new profession propelled into being by
the life-prolonging machines in the ICU. Employed by the hospital, Bramstedt functioned somewhat like an informal judge,
setting out and applying the rules when families, patients, and
medical staff were at odds. She was the arbiter when a family like mine found itself unexpectedly powerless in the face of
advanced medicine.

Most of her consults involved much more extreme power

struggles than ours between doctors and families over how to treat—or stop treating—desperately ill patients in intensive care, ravaged by deadly infections and kept alive with drugs, feeding tubes, respirators, and dialysis. She had her work cut out for her. In the ICU, there was no such thing as natural death, and few were comfortable with the timed event that had taken its place. Half the time, doctors wanted to keep going when families wanted to let go, and half the time, families—especially, but not only, African-American families—wanted to keep going when doctors wanted to quit. Sometimes doctors ignored advance directives from patients and even ripped them out of the charts. Sometimes a family would balk at implanting a feeding tube in a demented relative, only to hear a doctor say something like, "Nobody starves to death on my watch." Sometimes doctors complied when a long-estranged son or daughter—commonly referred to in hospitals as "The Nephew from Peoria"—flew in at the last minute and insisted that everything be done, even things that doctors and other family members thought were torturous, wasteful, and hopeless. When fragmented families collided with a fragmented medical system, the results could be disastrous.

An undercurrent of realistic worry ran through medical staff, administrators, and the in-house department, usually headed by an attorney, known as Risk Management. In a handful of extreme cases scattered across the country, distraught husbands and fathers had entered ICUs with guns and disconnected half-dead children from respirators or shot comatose wives in the head. On the other hand, if too much morphine was given, or too little done to try to save a life, a Nephew from Peoria might sue for negligence, or a local district attorney might even consider charges of manslaughter. A single unnecessarily prolonged intensive care death could cost a hospital well over $300,000—money not recovered from Medicare, which usually paid a lump sum based on the patient's diagnosis, no matter what the hospital's costs. The families, meanwhile, were often in shock: staggering to absorb reams of data from rotating casts of stranger-specialists who each zeroed in on a single organ and did not seem to talk to one another; fearful of death; ignorant of the limits of medicine; guilt stricken and religiously conflicted about ending life support; agonized by relatives' suffering; and hoping against hope.

In bland, untidy conference rooms edging the ICU, specialists asked families they'd never previously met to assent to the removal of life support, and spouses and children pondered questions—spiritual, legal, and medical—they rarely considered before tragedy hit. Did they have the right to say no to a doctor? To force a doctor to continue treatment? Was it God's will to do everything possible to prolong a life, no matter how much someone beloved was suffering? Was it suicide to refuse medical care? Was it murder not to give it? Was it a sin? And how were they to decide when the people they loved could no longer speak for themselves?

Out of this ongoing moral and logistical chaos, in which patients' families often felt disempowered, bioethicists like Bramstedt had created a semblance of order based on the philosophical and legal traditions of the West. She had read St. Augustine's teachings forbidding suicide and euthanasia and St. Thomas Aquinas's hair-splitting formulation of the principle of *double effect,* which allows a doctor to give a dying person morphine to relieve pain as long as the known side effect—hastened death—is not the motivating factor. She knew that Pope Pius XII declared in 1957 that good Catholics did not have to prolong their lives using *extraordinary means,* such as respirators. She had read the 1976 decision by the New Jersey Supreme Court, which quoted Aquinas and Pius XII when it permitted the devout Catholic parents of Karen Ann Quinlan to order the removal of the respirator from their daughter, who'd been in a persistent vegetative state since collapsing into unconsciousness at a party a year earlier, after consuming alcohol and valium. Bramstedt had studied the pioneering 1976 California statute that first validated the living will, inspired by the Quinlan case and passed the same year over the opposition of the Catholic Church, the American Medical Association, and the California ProLife Council.

She knew that a watershed 1990 U.S. Supreme Court decision, *Cruzan v. State of Missouri,* had further expanded—within limits—a patient's constitutional right to refuse medical treatment. Nancy Cruzan, a young Missouri woman who worked in a cheese factory, had been resuscitated by paramedics who found her facedown in a ditch, not breathing, after a one-vehicle car crash on the way home from a bar. By the time the U.S. Supreme Court heard her case, Cruzan had spent seven years in a state nursing home in what one Supreme Court justice called "a twilight zone of suspended animation" and a Missouri appeals court justice called "a living hell." Her parents (like the Quinlans, devout Catholics) sought to remove the feeding tube that kept her from dying, over the objections of the state of Missouri, which was then embroiled in a fierce political war over abortion. The Supreme Court affirmed that patients had the right to refuse any medical treatment, and that a feeding tube was, indeed, a medical treatment. But it also declared that the State of Missouri had an absolute and legitimate interest in the "preservation of life," and that Cruzan's parents had to prove to the state's satisfaction that removing the tube was an expression of their daughter's wishes and not their own.

It was Bramstedt's job, in a secular, religiously diverse culture with no consensus on these issues, or even a common language, to thread the needle among conflicting sets of values: the patient's legal right to medical autonomy; the state's interest in preserving life; the religious values of the family; the hospital's interest in avoiding a lawsuit; and the doctor's Hippocratic obligations to act out of "beneficence"—usually defined as doing more, not less—and not to assist in suicide or mercy killing. It was she who reassured families and doctors that it was morally and legally okay to deploy treatments that gave comfort while withholding treatments that prolonged the agony of death.

Despite more than twenty years of complaints by disempowered families over the brutal, unsanctified nature of death in the ICU, conflicts there remained the bread and butter of Bramstedt's ethics consults. But she had recently recognized a subtler new problem, one directly bearing on our family's dilemma.

Before becoming a bioethicist, Bramstedt had been a quality engineer for Guidant, then the third-largest U.S. maker of pacemakers and implantable cardiac defibrillators. (Defibrillators are advanced cardiac devices, more sophisticated than a pacemaker; they reboot the heart with a powerful shock when it races uncontrollably or falls into quivering arrhythmias.) The pacemaker and the defibrillator, Bramstedt told me, were creating ethical problems at the end of life, years after they were first put in. I took a breath.

"These devices are seen as simple and low-tech," she said. "You don't need to crack the chest. You toss them in and you go. But because cardiologists are so much into lifesaving, they don't think about the flip side of the coin. These devices are life-support technologies, which means the time will come when they need to be turned off."

Defibrillators, she went on, sometimes shocked patients unnecessarily, and when they did, patients felt as if they'd been kicked in the chest by a horse. If not deactivated, they could repeatedly shock people during their death agonies. Pacemakers, Bramstedt said, were more morally ambiguous. They might prolong life, but they didn't cause pain the way defibrillators or respirators did, and they often improved what she called "quality of life."

I took another breath. My father was not in a state of suspended animation like Nancy Cruzan. He could still eat his own breakfast. But he'd spent a whole weekend brushing his teeth. He dirtied his pants and felt ashamed. He could no longer take a walk on his own. Wasn't his life a sort of living hell? And what about my mother's?

There was, Bramstedt continued, little open discussion among cardiologists, and no consensus, about the legality and morality of turning off cardiac devices. But they were often deactivated just the same. In 2008, Bramstedt, working with a cardiologist, an internist, and a statistician from the Mayo Clinic, conducted an anonymous Web-based survey of 787 nurses, doctors, and device-company representatives who were members of the Heart Rhythm Society, a cardiology professional association. Eighty-seven percent reported they had been involved in requests to deactivate a cardiac device in a terminally ill patient. Of those, 92 percent had personally deactivated a defibrillator and 76 percent, a pacemaker. Many said they were less comfortable with deactivating pacemakers, which weren't seen as medically burdensome, than with deactivating defibrillators, which dramatically worsened quality of death. A fifth had refused a request to deactivate a pacemaker, and 11 percent considered pacemaker deactivation a form of euthanasia.

The problem, Bramstedt went on, was set in motion when the devices first went in. Patients should be informed *then,* she said, how long their devices would last, and that the time might come when they wished to have them turned off. That could be done painlessly, she said in an aside, without surgery.

That was news to me.

*   *   *

I made more calls and discovered that a white ceramic device, functioning like a TV remote and shaped like the wands that children use to blow bubbles, could be placed around the hump beneath my father's collarbone. Someone could press a few buttons and the electrical pulses that ran down the pacemaker's spiraled wires to his heart would slow until they were no longer effective. My father's heart would probably not stop. It would just return to its old, slow rhythm. If his aging heart had deteriorated since the pacemaker was put in, he might die within weeks. If he were unlucky, he might linger for months.

If we did nothing, his pacemaker would not stop for years.

Like the tireless charmed brooms that bedeviled the sorcerer's apprentice in Disney's *Fantasia*, the pacemaker would prompt my father's heart to beat after he became too demented to speak, sit up, or eat. It would briefly keep his heart twitching after he drew his last breath. If he were buried, it would keep sending electrical signals to his inert, dead heart in the coffin. If he were cremated, it would have to be cut from his chest first, to prevent it from exploding and damaging the walls or hurting an attendant.

I thought about the Cruzan case. If a feeding tube was medical treatment, wasn't a pacemaker? Surely my mother and I, as my father's "designated health care surrogates," had the legal and moral right to request its deactivation. It sounded eminently reasonable. But it didn't feel that way.

When my father had his first stroke, I knew at once my parents' world had been struck by lightning. Now I understood that the pacemaker had equally cleaved their world. *For the want of a nail, the horseshoe was lost; for the want of the horse, the rider was lost; for the want of the rider, the battle was lost; for the want of the battle, the kingdom was lost. And all for the want of a horseshoe nail.* If only my mother had asked for my opinion. If only I'd flown home. If only I'd known what to ask when I got there. If only my mother hadn't hidden her angst so skillfully and groomed my father so perfectly that he looked more functional than he was to Dr. Rogan, and she less desperate. If only someone had asked my father—who only a year later said he was "living too long"—whether he wanted to live to be ninety. Yet whom could I blame?

I made more calls. I learned that in an ideal world, doctors told their patients about the pros, cons, and alternatives to any proposed medical treatment. I learned that the pacemaker could have been avoided altogether if the hernia surgery had been performed another way, using a local anesthetic less risky to the heart. I learned we could have signed a waiver accepting the risks. I learned that the surgeon could have hooked my father's heart up to a temporary external pacemaker—a procedure that a leading cardiac surgeon told me was perfectly safe— and removed it after the hernias were sewn up and my father safely out of the recovery room.

I would raise these options years later with my father's cardiologist and surgeon. They were nonplussed. Said the surgeon, "Your father was still pretty together back then. It's hard to envision a scenario where you'd say, 'I've got to get that hernia fixed but don't worry about his heart!'" Said the cardiologist, "When one has a pretty solid indication for a permanent pacemaker, you don't usually do that [use a temporary device]. That's a risky situation versus a fairly minor procedure and a permanent solution." In any case, Dr. Rogan said, "Everyone takes for granted that it's the family care physician who really acts as a quarterback."

And where was Dr. Fales? Why did Medicare reward Dr. Aranow and Dr. Rogan far better for doing the procedure than it would have Dr. Fales for making a reasoned argument against it? "I spend forty-five minutes thinking through the problem, and I get seventy-five to a hundred bucks," Dr. Fales said when next we spoke. "Someone spends forty-five minutes putting in a pacemaker and is paid six times as much."

Why had "informed consent" for what Bramstedt defined as a miniaturized form of life support consisted of nothing more than a brief meeting with Dr. Aranow, at which my father had obediently affixed his wavering, spider-like signature to a ritual form whose checked boxes described only the generic risks of minor surgery? And what were we to do now?

I called my mother and told her that my father's pacemaker could be painlessly deactivated. She listened in silence. Years later I discovered that not long after our talk, she e-mailed a close friend in England and told her that I seemed to want to just get rid of my father.

That was where things stood when I found myself kneeling a month later on a meditation bench in a spacious hall among the dripping scrub oaks of northern California. A bell rang. I bowed to the Buddhas and headed for the door. The rain was beating its way down the square copper drainpipes as I moved slowly under my umbrella, in the silent company of others, down to the dining room. I'd arrived at Spirit Rock Meditation Center consumed by worry and obsession, furious about the pacemaker and sick of nagging my mother to get help. The inner microphone had been taken over by voices I barely noticed in my daily life: *You're not productive. You don't make enough money. Your house is a mess. Your man isn't good enough. You're letting your parents down.*

That evening, the rain stopped. The only sound I could hear in the meditation hall was the *ribbit* of a frog somewhere outside in the creek. My face softened like melting wax. My lips let go of their habitual tight line. Instead of coping with the debris on the surface of my mind, I was reveling in the peace below: the gentle rhythm of my breathing, the beating of my heart. It was as though I'd dropped down a dark well.

A man behind me cleared his throat. I stayed calm. In my right shoulder, nerves fired and faded in response, like a bright lace of phosphorescence stirred up by an oar in night water.

Earlier that day, our meditation teacher had suggested we avoid what she called the "Second Arrow." In a classic sutra, the Buddha had said that if someone shoots you in the foot, don't pick up the bow and shoot yourself in the foot again. Don't make your suffering worse, in other words, by arguing with what's so. That's a Second Arrow. Accept pain. Don't criticize yourself, or others, for feeling pain: that is a Second Arrow. Don't regret what cannot be changed, or try to predict what cannot be known. By throwing their complex machinery into the path of death, my father's doctors had shot my parents with a Second Arrow. And by trying too hard to shield my parents from suffering, I might be shooting myself—and them—with a Second Arrow as well.

CHAPTER 12

THE BUSINESS OF LIFESAVING

On the idealistic and hopeful day in 1958 when the forty-three-year-old Swedish ice-skater and businessman Arne Larsson was given the world's first fully implantable pacemaker, few in the worlds of business, engineering, or medicine foresaw a time when there would be a need or a market for hundreds of thousands more. Potential customers seemed at first glance few: a handful of "blue babies" and adults emerging from pioneering heart surgeries with unintended cardiac damage, and another handful of fatally ill people like Larsson who got dizzy and fainted multiple times a day because their hearts failed to maintain normal beats.

Things were about to change. Two years after Larsson's surgery, the pacemaker moved out of the hands of tinkerers and onto small assembly lines. By the end of December 1960, Medtronic's cofounder Earl Bakken—who'd been persuaded by a Lutheran minister when he was a teenager to turn his inventiveness away from tasers and toward helping people and who did not even mention "profit" in his company's original mission statement—had taken orders for fifty pacemakers, priced at $375 each.

In 1961, Bakken bought the licensing rights to a fully implantable pacemaker similar to Arne Larsson's, designed by the American inventor Wilson Greatbatch in a converted barn behind his house in Buffalo, New York. Sales were slow at first. In 1962, Medtronic lost $144,000. The next year, when U.S. health care spending was 5.3 percent of gross domestic product (GDP), and the average American life span was close to seventy, Medtronic sold only twelve hundred pacemakers and edged barely into the black. The start-up was so starved for capital that Bakken considered selling it to the Mallory Battery Company, but the deal fell through after the Arthur D. Little consulting company estimated that only ten thousand people worldwide would ever need pacemakers. Then, in 1965, Medicare—the Great Society insurance program bitterly opposed by the American Medical Association (AMA) and championed, like the 911 system, by the heart attack survivor President Lyndon B. Johnson—was established. It approved the pacemaker for reimbursement the following year for any American over the age of sixty-five with a medical need for one, and Earl Bakken's world changed.

In the first full year of Medicare reimbursement, when health care consumed only 5.9 percent of GDP, Medtronic sold seven thousand four hundred pacemakers, six times as many as it had three years before. It made a profit of nearly $308,000. Two years later, in 1968, it reported annual sales of $10 million and profits of more than $1 million. By 1970, health care spending was consuming 7.2 percent of GDP, and Medtronic's annual sales had more than doubled, to $22 million. Pacemakers had become the company's cash cow.

The atmosphere in what would later be nicknamed "Medical Alley"—Minnesota's cluster of high-tech medical start-ups—soon rivaled that of the nascent semiconductor industry near Stanford University in northern California's Santa Clara Valley. In small towns on the outskirts of Minneapolis and St. Paul, engineers, visionaries, and salespeople rented offices; wooed venture capitalists; invented, borrowed, and stole innovative technologies; and sued one another for patent infringement and theft of intellectual property. Members of a new breed of sales-man—part electrical engineer, part medical paraprofessional, and part Willy Loman—fanned out across the country, enter-ing operating rooms dressed in scrubs just like doctors, to show eager but ignorant physicians how to implant the new devices. Big corporations bought out small companies. Initial public offerings showcased shares that doubled in price within hours of hitting the stock market and stayed high.

Four Medtronic engineers and salesmen, frustrated with Earl Bakken's cautious approach to technological innovation, left his company to manufacture a slimmer pacemaker also designed by Wilson Greatbatch but powered by a longer-lasting, hermeti-cally sealed lithium battery. (The earlier models had mercury-zinc batteries, which released small amounts of hydrogen gas and lasted only a year or two before needing replacement.) The start-up, Cardiac Pacemakers, Inc., was financed with $50,000 in bank loans and $450,000 in venture capital. Its pacemaker was barely more than a prototype, and at first its salesmen had nothing to show doctors but a wooden mock-up. It had almost no sales in 1972, its first year.

Four years later, with health care now consuming 8.4 per-cent of GDP, and the average American life span creeping up toward seventy-three, Cardiac Pacemakers had $47 million in sales. "The profit margins were beautiful in those days," said one of the company's founders, Manuel Villafaña, a colorful former Medtronic salesman born in the South Bronx who'd earlier introduced Medtronic pacemakers to doctors in South America and Europe. Cardiac Pacemakers' after-tax profits were 20 percent. Two years later, its founders sold the company to the Eli Lilly pharmaceutical company for $127 million. Renamed Guidant, it would later branch into coronary stents and other cardiac hardware and become the world's third-largest manufacturer of cardiac-surgery devices—and would employ Katrina Bramstedt, who later became a bioethicist. In 2004, it was sold to Boston Scientific and Abbott Laboratories for $27.2 billion.

Spin-offs begat spin-offs. Manuel Villafaña left Cardiac Pacemakers to found St. Jude Medical, Inc., which developed and promoted a new heart valve made of stone-hard pyrolytic carbon, a major advance over the bulkier metal and plastic ball-and-ring models, prone to clotting, then being used by surgeons such as Dwight Harken at Peter Bent Brigham Hospital in Boston. The St. Jude valve became the most commonly used in the world; in one of its early years, after-tax profits hit 48 percent. St. Jude would use those accumulated profits a couple of decades later to buy a thriving international pacemaker company called Pacesetter, part of the German industrial and health behemoth Siemens, which had earlier swallowed Elema-Schönander, the Swedish company whose inventors saved Arne Larsson's life.

The secret to success from the first was a guaranteed market and close-to-guaranteed prices. Unlike the tightly controlled, government-run variants of universal health care then being pioneered in many European countries, Medicare functioned more like a government-funded insurance company. Thanks to intense lobbying from the AMA, it was never given authority to negotiate bulk discounts, to request bids for standardized models, to second-guess a doctor's decision, to control prices, or otherwise to interfere with what the AMA called the "doctor-patient relationship." In the United States, a handful of pacemaker companies, enjoying a near monopoly, essentially set prices. Individual doctors decided independently who needed the devices and billed Medicare their "usual and customary" fees. Hospitals provided operating rooms and ancillary services, exercised little control over the doctors who used them, and billed Medicare separately. Medicare simply paid. Thanks to this unique financial structure—a griffin-like hybrid with neither the marketplace checks and balances of capitalism nor the top-down government controls of socialism—pacemakers and other emerging medical technologies were delivered practically cost-free to the hospital, surgeon, and patient. The system had no brakes.

As profits grew and sales forces expanded in Medical Alley, the thinking and practice of many cardiologists across the country changed. In its pioneering days, the pacemaker was regarded as a specialized lifesaver for a handful of otherwise healthy people with fatal disturbances in heart rhythm. After Medicare, as the devices improved technologically and inserting them became simple and profitable, the rationale changed. Doctors began inserting them to improve "quality of life" in a much larger pool of older people with minor heart arrhythmias. They next began inserting them on a "just in case" basis in relatively healthy people whose hearts were slowing down naturally with age but who had no symptoms at all. People like my father.

In 1974, a Columbia Medical School cardiologist named Irene Ferrer, a sister of the actor Mel Ferrer, argued that "periodic or sustained sinus bradycardia [that is, a slow heartbeat] can no longer go unchallenged, even if asymptomatic." Pacemakers, she said, should be implanted on a "prophylactic" [preventive] basis, particularly in patients in a broad new diagnostic category called "sick sinus syndrome," characterized by a variety of modest disturbances in the heart rhythm revealing themselves on newer, ever-more-sensitive diagnostic machines. Pacemaker

implantations doubled year by year. The guiding principles of
the day were maximum promotion and maximum treatment.

Behind the scenes, meanwhile, Medicare—which paid for
about 85 percent of pacemaker insertions and thus was primar-
ily responsible for the explosive growth of the industry—was
changing the shape of American medicine. Medicare's framers had hoped to provide better medical care for the elderly.
They did. The average life span increased from sixty-five in
1940 to seventy-one in 1970. Deaths from heart disease fell.
But because Medicare mimicked the fee-for-service structure
of existing private insurance plans, it paid better for procedures
than for time. It starved doctors who provided hands-on primary
care and overrewarded specialists who churned out procedures.
Pay for primary care doctors was so poor that some of them refused
to take Medicare patients at all. Doctors peddled their wares on a
piecework basis; communication among them became haphaz-
ard; thinking was often short-term; nobody made money when
medical interventions were declined; and nobody was in charge
except the marketplace.

Fueled not only by Medicare but also by private health insurance, doctors' average incomes quintupled—from $50,000 a year
in 1940 in 2011 dollars to nearly $250,000 in 1970. Most of the
increase went to specialists. Doctors flocked to where the money
was: by 1969, there were nearly three specialists for each primary
care doctor in America. When Medicare approved coverage for
routine colonoscopies, gastroenterology incomes rose, and so did
the number of gastroenterologists.

Newly enlarged high-rise hospitals—technological palaces
fueled by private insurance and by federal dollars for research,
construction, and patient care—were built in cities across the
country. In their shadows often lay neighborhoods of the impoverished and the working poor, served, if at all, by a dwindling
pool of underpaid and low-status internists and family doc-

tors who maintained close emotional relationships with their patients throughout their lifetimes. Among those who suffered most, along with the poor, were the chronically ill and elderly of all classes: those with problems that couldn't be fixed, who most needed the soft technologies of thoughtful, old-fashioned doctoring; advice on lifestyle and adaptation; and the time-consuming hands-on attention of a general practitioner. Despite the best intentions of its framers, Medicare's payment structure punished doctors who practiced the Slow Medicine the elderly often needed and rewarded those on the hard-tech cutting edge.

Cardiac hypermarketing, meanwhile, grew so outrageous that it drew attention outside the hermetically sealed worlds of the operating room and Medical Alley. In what turned out to be the first of repeating waves of scandals similar to those in the pharmaceutical industry, witnesses told a Senate subcommittee in 1981 that some doctors were deliberately performing unnecessary pacemaker implantations in return for device industry kickbacks. Sales reps at one pacemaker company—a company, as it happened, with a terrible product-safety record—gave their most "productive" doctors free stays at the company hunting lodge and on the company yacht. Others hired the comedian George Burns and the cheerleaders for the Dallas Cowboys to regale doctors at free dinners and parties. "In all my twenty years experience in the medical sales field, I have never seen a business so dirty, so immensely profitable, and so absent normal competitive price controls as this one," one former salesman told the Senate subcommittee.

The subcommittee issued a tough report entitled "Fraud, Waste and Abuse in the Medicare Pacemaker Industry." The FBI investigated. Medicare drastically revamped its payment system in an attempt to get a handle on costs. In 1983, several executives of Siemens-Pacesetter, Inc. (the pacemaker company later acquired by St. Jude, which made my father's pacemaker)

pled guilty and its former CEO pled nolo contendere to federal charges that they'd paid kickbacks to doctors for implanting
pacemakers. They were given suspended sentences and fined.

Some troubled cardiologists—often those paid salaries by
universities rather than earning a living in private practice—had
growing doubts about where the whole enterprise was leading.
At a cardiology conference in Manhattan devoted to the elimi-
nation of fatal heart attacks, Henry Greenberg, the director of a
hospital coronary care unit, delivered a contrarian and prescient
paper called "In Praise of Sudden Death." He'd informally polled
his cardiologist friends and their families, he said, and "not one
wished anything but a sudden, unexpected exit while in the pink
of health. There were not even any votes for a classic deathbed scene, with the family gathered." The preferred age for this
death, he said, was around eighty. "We all want to live to the
fullest extent of our capacity as a sapient being capable of joy
and delight, but at the proper time life can be quickly and gently
rounded with a sleep," he told his cardiology colleagues in 1982:

> What if we are fully successful in the purpose of our gath-
> ering? Will we devoutly wish for a new risk factor to call
> into play as we see memory slipping as our dotage arises?
> Will we avoid physicians and hospitals for routine ailments
> because we are afraid that unacceptable illnesses will be
> prolonged interminably?

In the aftermath of the pacemaker scandal, a committee
appointed by the American College of Cardiology wrote a set
of clinical guidelines in 1984 intended to discourage overtreatment. On a logic that boiled down to "if it ain't broke, don't
fix it," the committee advised against implanting the devices in
patients with no troubling physical symptoms and no sign of disease beyond slightly irregular cardiograms, slow heartbeats, or

vague diagnoses such as sick sinus syndrome. Over the next five years, pacemaker implantations in Medicare patients dropped by 25 percent. But the basic pattern—maximum promotion, the creeping expansion of diagnoses for which pacemakers and other cardiac devices were supposedly warranted, disguised gratuities to cardiologists, and cat-and-mouse games with Medicare—did not end. No matter how Medicare tried to change its rules and tighten the spigot, money continued to flood into the device companies, and like water seeking its own level, some of that money trickled down to cardiologists. By 1987, the median income of cardiovascular surgeons was $271,555, while most primary care doctors earned considerably less than $100,000.

One former Medtronic sales rep told me that in the 1980s he was sent to a three-day course in fine wines, all the better to wine, dine, and knowledgeably converse with the upscale cardiologists who were his sales prospects. In the early 1990s, one of pacemaking's pioneers, a respected university-based cardiac surgeon, saw how far things had gone wrong when he flew from the east coast to Los Angeles to supervise the placement of a pacemaker in his mother-in-law, who was then in her early nineties. "I went out there on a Saturday to Cedars Sinai, I guess in February," said the east coast surgeon, who asked to remain anonymous. "It was a very quiet day, and the surgeon and I were sort of waiting around. It turned out we were waiting for the sales rep, and finally he arrived. The doctor put in the pacemaker adequately, and the sales rep handed the surgeon a package and left. The surgeon opened it in front of me, seemingly not at all embarrassed; it was a nice gold wristwatch, as a present."

Time passed. Things changed. Things stayed the same. The number of transistors in a typical pacemaker grew from only two to more than four million. U.S. health care costs kept rising, to nearly double those in some European countries, without a corresponding gain in health. In 2003, the year my father got his device, when health care was consuming 15.9 percent of GDP and the average American life span had risen to seventy-seven, a Medicare study found that medical device companies were enjoying average net profit margins of nearly 20 percent. It was, the *New York Times* pointed out, more than twice the average for all other companies in the S&P 500. Cardiac surgery was so profitable that many hospitals relied on it to subsidize their emergency rooms and other money-losing departments and ran full-page ads in major newspapers to attract new customers. Cardiologists published a flurry of journal articles about successful surgeries in patients over eighty and over ninety. Device-related heart surgeries alone in 2003 cost Medicare nearly $15 billion.

By then, there were all kinds of devices: stents, little cage-like tubes to prop open clogged arteries; drug-coated stents, less prone to clogging than bare metal ones; external heart pumps like the one that would later be attached to former Vice President Dick Cheney, each one costing Medicare more than $500,000. There were chemically pickled and sterilized heart valves taken from human cadavers and from pigs, and delicate bionic valves hand sewn in Southern California factories by Vietnamese-American and Cambodian-American women working with the sterilized heart tissue of cows.

In May 2003, Michael N. Weinstein, a senior analyst at J.P. Morgan, called the cardiac device business "an area of tremendous interest." Medical devices of all sorts had become a $170 billion global industry, and cardiac devices alone generated $14 billion in worldwide sales. Weinstein's "top pick," he told an interviewer for the *New York Times*'s Market Insight column, "is St. Jude Medical. They are a play on the cardiac rhythm market."

The market was not pleased, however, in the spring of 2006 when Medicare proposed yet another change in the formulas under which it reimbursed hospitals, in hopes of reducing payments for implanted devices and raising payments for under-compensated services like stroke care. Payments for pacemaker surgeries were expected to drop by about 13 percent, defibrillators by 25 percent, and stents by 33 percent. AdvaMed, the device industry's primary voice in Washington, pushed back. In April, AdvaMed hired two former health care staffers from the House Ways and Means Committee and another who'd once worked in health policy for Senator Ted Kennedy.

Over the next few months, AdvaMed spent $1 million on what its chief called "inside the Beltway advertising and extensive media outreach, 'grass tops' advocacy efforts, and intense lobbying of key House and Senate Members." It created a photo exhibit on Capitol Hill featuring enthusiastic patients such as Reagan administration official Michael Deaver, who had an artificial knee; former Olympic skater Bonnie Blair, who'd benefited from an implanted anti-incontinence surgical device; and a former NBA basketball player who had a pacemaker. It held a press conference featuring the heads of two nonprofit, apparently grassroots, groups—the Sudden Cardiac Arrest Association, a defibrillator-promoting group funded mainly by the cardiac device industry; and the Society for Women's Health Research, which got most of its grants from big medical players, including the Medtronic Foundation and Boston Scientific.

What went unremarked was the eternal background music of Washington. The makers of pharmaceuticals and medical supplies constitute one of the capital's three biggest lobbies, rivaling the defense industry and Wall Street. In 2006, AdvaMed, the Big Three pacemaker companies, and other medical technology and supply companies spent at least $27 million on lobbying Medicare, the Food and Drug Administration, Congress, and other parts of the federal government. They contributed another $1.5 million to federal political campaigns.

The money and attention were well spent. After two hundred members of the House and Senate from both parties wrote to Medicare questioning the proposed cutbacks, its top administrator, Mark McClellan, said he had taken the objections "to heart" and essentially gutted the plan, making changes that in the estimation of AdvaMed, recaptured $3 billion in at-risk sales revenues. Shares of Medtronic, St. Jude Medical, and Boston Scientific rose on the news.

Business as usual continued, and money continued to flow and drip from device companies to cardiologists. In 2007—the year that my father forgot the purpose of his dinner napkin—a registered nurse named Charles Donigian resigned from his job in the regional sales office of St. Jude Medical in St. Louis, Missouri, where he'd helped administer follow-up surveys of patients who'd been given pacemakers and defibrillators. Donigian said he resigned because he thought he'd soon be fired for refusing to bend ethical rules. He subsequently filed a lawsuit seeking damages under the federal law that protects whistleblowers.

In his suit, which the Justice Department later joined, Donigian said that St. Jude had essentially paid kickbacks to doctors who chose its products, in the form of what he called "sham fees for phony postmarket clinical research studies." In one study, St. Jude paid the doctors $2,000 per enrolled patient. The doctors mainly provided the names, Donigian claimed, while he and others at St. Jude did the paperwork as well as the doctors' Medicare billings.

St. Jude salesmen also gifted doctors with fishing trips to Canada, tickets to St. Louis Cardinals games, airline tickets to Las Vegas, and dinners at steak houses, Donigian said. One sales representative, he said, had an expense account of $250,000 a year, mainly to entertain and reward cardiologists. The corruption went both ways: one cardiac catheterization lab, he claimed, told St. Jude sales reps they expected a catered lunch for the entire office each time they implanted a St. Jude product.

Donigian said that St. Jude employees ghostwrote two research presentations summarizing the results of one cardiac follow-up study (the RARE trial), and paid one of the doctors named as a lead investigator to travel to the annual meeting of the Heart Rhythm Society, the cardiac device specialist's group, and present the findings in a scientific poster session in the exhibit hall as if they were his own.

Donigian said that St. Jude planned to spend $158 million on educational and career guidance programs for "fellows," young cardiologists training in electrophysiology, the subspecialty that manages cardiac devices. An internal marketing document estimated that each of the one hundred fellows who became a full-fledged electrophysiologist and conservatively prescribed St. Jude products could generate $2.7 million in device sales a year. After the Justice Department joined the case, St. Jude, without admitting wrongdoing, settled the lawsuit in early 2011 for $16 million, of which Donigian received $2.6 million. The Code of Business Conduct on the St. Jude Web site states that salespeople's gifts to doctors should not be "extravagant" or "beyond that which is customary," but those terms are not defined.

In 2008, a year after Donigian quit, the American College of Cardiology, the Heart Rhythm Society, and the American Heart Association issued the latest update of their treatment guidelines for pacemakers. The list of diagnoses for which they were strongly or mildly recommended had grown since the guidelines were first issued in 1984. The 1984 guidelines recommended pacemakers for fifty-six heart conditions. The 2008 guidelines recommended them for eighty-eight. The research backing the expansion was weak, with only 5 percent of the positive recommendations backed by medical research's "gold standard": multiple randomized double-blind studies. Most were based only on a consensus of "expert opinion." Of the seventeen cardiologists who wrote the 2008 guidelines, eleven received financing from cardiac-device makers or worked at institutions receiving it. Seven, due to the extent of their financial connections, were recused from voting on the guidelines they helped write.

This pattern—a paucity of scientific support and a plethora of industry connections—held across almost all cardiac treatment guidelines, said cardiologist Pierluigi Tricoci of Duke University and his coauthors in an article published in 2009 in the *Journal of the American Medical Association.* "Experts are as vulnerable to conflicts of interest as researchers are," they wrote, and added that the current cardiac-research agenda was "strongly influenced by industry's natural desire to introduce new products."

That desire would be on full display in the spring of 2011, two years after my father's death, when I parked in a municipal parking garage on Mission Street near the *San Francisco Chronicle,* my old newspaper, and walked toward the Moscone Convention Center, where the Heart Rhythm Society was holding its annual conference. It was a sunny, windy day in the South of Market district. The first thing that caught my eye was a fleet of black motorcycles repeatedly circling the block, each one towing a shiny black minitrailer bearing the logo of St. Jude Medical ("More Control! Less Risk!"). Towering above me on the side of a two-story building were five orange, turquoise, blue, and purple billboards, each bigger than a movie marquee, trumpeting the behemoth Medtronic's implantable cardiac defibrillators ("Fewer Shocks! MRI Access!"), its surgical tools for a heart procedure called cardiac ablation ("Inflation/Ablation!"), and its corporate logo ("Innovating for Life!"). A commercial white stretch limousine idled by the curbside, trolling for customers.

Outside the convention center, the sides of official shuttle buses were covered with company logos. Inside the hall were more logos—for Biosense, Johnson & Johnson, Siemens, Zoll, and Greatbatch—plastered on water coolers, on piles of complimentary tourist maps of San Francisco, on Internet access booths, and above laptop charging stations. A sign above the couches of the Infinity Circle where tired cardiologists checked their e-mail read, "Year Round Support: Infinite Gratitude: Heart Rhythm Society," followed by a list of its top corporate contributors, including Medtronic, Boston Scientific, St. Jude Medical, and Sanofi Aventis ("Because Health Matters"). All told, medical technology companies paid the Heart Rhythm Society $5.1 million—nearly a third of its $16.8 million annual budget—to rent exhibit booths and otherwise promote themselves to the more than three thousand physicians attending the four-day convention. This was the sea in which cardiologists swam.

St. Jude Medical, the maker of my father's device and the conference's third-biggest spender, paid $653,000, including $15,000 for ads on the risers of stairs, $45,000 for the privilege of hosting complimentary dinner seminars and other educational events for doctors in hotel banquet rooms, $55,000 to hang banners above stairways, $70,000 to put its logo on the cardiologists' hotel key cards, and $308,000 for exhibit booth space on the showroom floor. The company was on *Fortune*'s list of the world's most admired companies. It employed about thirteen hundred sales representatives and was a member of the Fortune 500, with a market capitalization of $13 billion.

Wearing my press badge and carrying the complimentary tote bag I was handed in the well-stocked press room, I walked into Moscone's huge underground commercial exhibit hall. It reminded me of a combination of a carnival midway, an auto showroom, and the largest Apple store on earth. Everywhere I looked, flat-screens glowed and pulsed, displaying loops of medical-technology advertising. The average American life span was now seventy-eight and a half, and health care was consuming 17.9 percent of America's GDP per year. Salesmen and saleswomen with expensive haircuts circled clutches of slim, vital doctors in sharp dark suits. Suspended above our heads in the hangar-like space were gigantic plastic signboards in whites and cool blues and greens, reading, "St. Jude Medical," "Medtronic," and "Biotronik: Excellence for Life."

A kind and handsome sales engineer at the St. Jude Medical booth—it wasn't a booth, really, it was at least four times the size of my living room—handed me a pacemaker much like the one Dr. Aranow had tucked into the pocket of skin beneath my late father's collarbone years before. It was flattish, roughly ovoid and encased in titanium, the color of dull silver. About the size of a pocket watch, it looked a little like a silver dollar that had been flattened on a railroad track. "St. Jude Medical, TM," was engraved on its side, along with the location of the factory where it was made: Sylmar, California. It fit into my palm.

I closed my hand around the tiny little machine that had saved many a life, made many a fortune, and led my family to so much unnecessary suffering.

CHAPTER 13

DEACTIVATION

In the spring of 2007, when my father was eighty-four, incontinent, wobbly, sleeping for hours during the day, and virtually confined to the house, Brian and I went to England on vacation. One day I took a bus alone to 21 Thorncliffe Road, the little brick and gray stone row house where my father told me stories in front of the fire when he was a student at Oxford and I was a little girl. I rang the bell. A young mother, a renter, let me take a look around the ground floor. It was much as I remembered it except for an updated kitchen: a scattering of children's toys, a few small rooms, and a strip of walled back garden that no longer sheltered an apple tree. When I got home, I sent my father a copy of the photo of me standing by our old front door. To my right, between our flagstone path and the neighbor's, was a low, unremarkable brick wall.

In May I opened an almost illegible letter, in miniature handwriting, the last my demented and partly blind father would
ever send me. I puzzled it out letter by letter and focused on the
few sentences I could fully decipher. This is exactly how it read.

Dear Katy,
   Thank you for the letter letter from Oxford. The old
adges from from the old old from Thorncliffe road is really
splendid remiddedid and other little made me me this letter made me me on still setle.
   I did that wall and sill when you were tiny thing.

I took out the photograph and looked at the brick wall. I
could remember my one-armed father, black-haired, strong
and whistling, building that wall on a Saturday morning in the
1950s: making a neat pile of his bricks, rigging up a horizon-
tal white string to keep his rows aligned, and troweling up his
cement on a plywood square.

   When your number when you were and I and it was.
   I see in the photgraph who took. I see. I made the lwit-
ing wrad and its its still up there.
   So it stands for all those years. Thank you for the toast
post. It really is a joy.
                                          all my love, Jeff.

Every day, my mother said, he lost yet another word, practical skill, or memory. Once he'd needed her care hour by hour.
Now he needed her supervision minute by minute. In her journal, she wrote of my father's "slow but progressing dementia. . . .
I am so weary of his problems and wish I had a life of my own."
Later I would learn that my father had reached stage five or six
of dementia's seven roughly sequential stages. It is a terminal ill-

ness, and in the seventh, final stage, people forget how to walk, smile, swallow, eat, or breathe. My mother had come round to my view of the pacemaker. "We all in the family wish," she wrote in her journal, "that the pacemaker had not been put in at all."

Meeting once a month at a coffee shop on Main Street and in one another's kitchens, my mother and three other Middletown women caring for impaired and dependent husbands had formed their own support group. One was a financial planner in her seventies still working full time to cover her husband's nursing-home bills. Another was caring for her husband, a retired artist with Parkinson's still living at home. The third was a college professor whose husband, also at home, had early-onset Alzheimer's and could not speak. They and my mother exchanged tips on nursing homes and caregivers and adult day care programs and wept together after reading a journal article I sent my mother on ambiguous loss. One night they held a pot-luck at my mother's house, the women chatting volubly while those husbands who were still at liberty sat mutely or stood awkwardly and stared at one another.

I do not know exactly what led my mother to decide the time had come. But in the summer of 2007, during a routine cardiology appointment, she asked Dr. Rogan to deactivate the pacemaker. He said that she would need a court order declaring my father incompetent, and she passed the news on to me. When I asked her about her decision later, she said, "It was hard. I was doing for Jeff what I would have wanted him to do for me."

In answer to questions I posed him, Dr. Rogan would later write me a letter describing his shock at her request. He had previously worked as a critical-care doctor and had turned off pacemakers on deathbeds, he said. But in his eyes, my father's situation was different: he wasn't on the brink of dying. "Your father walked in on his own accord and answered simple questions appropriately," he wrote me. "Your mother wanted it turned off. I told her I doubted [his heart had] any significant intrinsic rhythm and that turning [the pacemaker] off might well result in him dying on the spot, to which your mother said, and I will never forget, 'Good, that is what I want.' He made no indication that is what *he* wanted and he was competent at the time to my knowledge."

This was my mother's turning point. When my father was vigorous and lucid, she regarded medicine as her wily ally in a lifelong campaign to keep old age, sickness, and death at bay. Now ally and foe exchanged masks. Medicine looked more like the enemy, and death the friend. The next time she took my father to the internist, Dr. Fales told her quietly, "You don't have to do everything they say."

She cancelled an appointment with my father's neurologist, refused another scan of my father's brain to see if he'd had more strokes, and declined to put him on Aricept for his dementia or on Coumadin, an antistroke drug that carries a risk of uncontrolled bleeding and requires close monitoring and limiting one's intake of dark green vegetables. When Dr. Rogan asked her to bring my father in for two separate heart tests, each requiring hours of fasting, she agreed to only one. She cancelled all further appointments with Dr. Rogan and agreed to only two telephone pacemaker checks a year. "I take responsibility for whatever," she wrote. "Enough of all this overkill! It's killing me! Talk about quality of life—what about mine?"

Meanwhile, I was spending my Wednesday evenings in a conference room at the Merchant's Exchange Building in downtown San Francisco, listening to people who worked mostly in high-tech give short, extemporaneous speeches and clapping enthusiastically for them at all the right moments, as they did for me. At the suggestion of my brother Jonathan, who'd once been a car salesman, I'd enrolled in a Dale Carnegie course in effective human relations and communication. I was now managing my parents' investments and trying to plan for their uncertain future, and after six years of long-distance caregiving, I felt isolated and stale. I hoped that the training would teach me to get along better with Brian's sons and to make a good impression on the editors I was courting in a shrinking magazine market. I did not tell my mother: *Dale Carnegie* had long been my father's contemptuous shorthand for glad-handing, commercially driven, overly positive American insincerity.

Many of my fellow students at Dale Carnegie were younger than I. Some were engineers born in India, Vietnam, or Europe and working here on H-1B visas for software and cell-phone companies. Each week we practiced remembering and using people's first names ("the sweetest sound in the English language!"); being generous with praise; and asking others about their hobbies, pets, and children but not their politics, sexuality, or religion. We were told to "cooperate with the inevitable." We learned that the only way to win an argument was to avoid one. We learned to say, "If I were in your shoes, I'd feel exactly the same way." We learned not to criticize, condemn, or complain. After the course was over, I got a quick haircut at a San Francisco Supercuts and flew east.

The weather in Connecticut was sharp and clear. Toni picked me up at the airport in my mother's white Camry, and we drove to my parents' home on Pine Street as the sun set. My mother opened the door; my father, sitting blankly in the living room, did not get up, and for the first time ever, did not smile when I kissed him. I told my mother how nice the house looked and remarked on a whorl of dried twigs she'd twisted into a wreath and hung on the fireplace wall above a narrow, bleached horse's skull she found long ago in the Maine woods and a copy of an

Albrecht Dürer engraving of a horse's head. She was wearing, as always, a pair of silver hoop earrings she'd bought long before in Vermont. Her white hair was neatly gathered at the nape of her neck, camouflaging the bald spot on her crown, and she looked tired, but not too tired to cast an assessing eye over my hair and clothes. I was in baggy blue jeans, white athletic socks, running shoes, a no-iron white shirt, and a dark-blue fleece jacket. My dyed brown hair, newly cut, ballooned over my forehead in a bulbous helmet. As she and I twittered through our first hellos, my father said little, beyond an occasional, "I don't know what you're talking about!" or "What are we doing now?" Within minutes, my mother and I were acting as if he weren't there.

My father's main expression now was one of perpetual confusion. When dinnertime came, he looked anxiously at my mother and would not move toward the kitchen until she gave him her nod. She was his true north now: he did not like to have her out of his sight.

I enjoyed watching him eat. There I saw a competence that had disappeared elsewhere. He reminded me of an ancient parrot, slow, silent, and deliberate, using his thumb and forefinger like a beak to methodically chase the last leaf of lettuce around his plate. My mother cleared away the remainder of the chicken breasts she'd sautéed in butter and finished with shallots and a dash of vermouth. I handed him a glass of water and put in front of him the square blue china dish holding his pills and vitamins. He picked up the glass and poured the water into the pill dish and watched gravely as water overflowed onto the table and floor. He stopped only when I took the glass from his hand. From then on I would hide the water glass behind my back, hand him the pills, tell him to put them in his mouth, and then hand him the water glass and tell him, like a dog, to drink.

As I sponged up the water, I noted my father could no longer rise easily from his chair—a warning sign, I would later learn, of looming total debility. He grabbed the edge of the table with his thumb and forefinger and rocked his body forward and back, oscillating perilously until he had enough momentum to thrust himself upright. I wondered how long it would be before he became bedridden, and how we would handle him then. He wobbled and tottered. His grip, when I anxiously took his hand to shepherd him up the stairs, was still strong and warm. I could feel his life force, still coursing. Wounded as he was, he was still emotional ballast for my mother and for me.

Once our procession arrived at the upstairs bathroom door, I turned away, leaving him and my mother to their highly taxing and to my mind, unnecessarily complex, bedtime ritual. My mother seemed fixated on the notion that thoroughly brushing, flossing, and water-picking my father's expensive dental implants, according to a strict protocol, still mattered.

The bathroom door closed behind them. Before heading down to the kitchen to wash the dishes, I paused at a bend in the stairs. Through the bathroom door and the thin Sheetrock walls, I could hear her shouting at him. There was a short silence and then a cry. My father was whimpering like an exhausted, demoralized, and beaten child. I will never forget that cry. Later my mother would admit, in passing, that there had been times when she "clouted" him. (She was not alone: 5 to 10 percent of long-term caregivers for people with severe dementia admit to similar physical abuse, often out of depression, exhaustion, and frustration.)

In her fifties, after she survived surgery, radiation, and breast cancer, my mother liked to say that sometimes the worst things that happen turn out to be the best things. She believed, as did Ernest Hemingway, that the world breaks all of us and afterward some are strong in the broken places, and that she was among the strong. She did not say that now. "Some griefs augment the heart, enlarge. Some stunt," wrote the poet Jane Hirshfield. My father's decline had at first forced my mother to become more accepting, and me, more openly loving. Now I stood paralyzed as caregiving destroyed my mother's moral fiber and corroded her soul.

When bioethicists debate life-prolonging technologies, their moral and physical effects on people like my mother rarely enter the calculus. But during the last year of my father's life, Ohio State University released a study of the DNA of family members who were looking after relatives with dementia. It showed that the ends of their chromosomes, called telomeres, had degraded enough to reflect a four- to eight-year shortening of life span. By that reckoning, for every year the pacemaker gave my damaged father, it took from my mother an equal year.

After breakfast the next morning, while I was dialing a home health care agency in West Hartford from the kitchen phone, my father appeared at the doorway, pointing downward with a troubled look. I herded him toward the downstairs bathroom, ignoring my mother as she insisted he didn't need to go, and continuing to ignore her as she shouted, "Go upstairs!" to the toilet with the special Toto rinsing attachment that automatically cleaned off his bottom. My father barely got onto the downstairs toilet in time to sit down. My mother entered the small space and pulled him up to clean off his bottom. He peed on the floor and sat down again to shit. I turned away, nearly retching, and ran upstairs, where I got my mother a clean, warm, wet washcloth. She was still shouting at my father as she took it. I put my hands gently on her shoulders, full of love and force, and called her by her first name, saying, "Val. Stop."

It was the first time I'd physically confronted her since I was a teenager and refused to let her slap me anymore. She turned to me in a fury, a poor, shrunken, horrible, exhausted, demoralized old lady. If she'd been forty years younger, she'd have "clouted" me. She dropped the washcloth and walked out of the bathroom in tears. And then the enigma that was their marriage once again blindsided me. My father—who by then had sixty years of practice in selectively tuning my mother out—caught my eye, shrugged, and gave me an amused, almost conspiratorial naughty-boy smile. *Oh Well!* he seemed to be saying. *What can you do? That's your mother for you!*

Once the drama was over and my mother had cleaned up the mess and gotten my father dressed, he took his customary seat in the living room in a heavy, untippable wrought-iron chair my mother had brought in from the garden since my last visit. There he sat for hours on his waterproof cushion, holding a book in his lap, not turning the pages, sometimes dozing, sometimes looking up to watch the leaves fall.

I made a great show of insisting my father come out on the deck with me, and as if it mattered, help me sweep away the dry leaves, eternally falling.

I had only one item on my agenda for my visit: getting my mother to hire more help. I had done the calculations: even with the most profligate hiring of aides, their money would last them three to five years. It was, as far as I could see, the only option. My mother would never put my father in a nursing home. I would never call an elder-abuse hotline. She'd tried an adult day care program recommended by her support group, but my father had become disoriented and disruptive and refused to go back. She reluctantly agreed to let me try to find someone to supplement Toni. "I know I need it," she wrote in her journal. "But I jib at my loss of privacy, and also a thought that I do it best."

When the young West African woman from the Nightingale's home health agency arrived for her first four-hour shift—their minimum—the silence was thick. My mother could not abide having a stranger in the house, even one who quietly read in the living room over the dinner hour. She had grown up witnessing the suffering of black servants at her own mother's hands in the formal, intimate cruelty of the old South Africa, and she bridled at any reminder of the place she'd fled. We were entering white water. The old rules no longer applied. If she didn't let go, we would drown.

At lunch, my mother had me turn my head from side to side. She said I needed to get that haircut fixed. And then, while my father napped, she asked me for the first time to help her get his pacemaker turned off. I was witnessing a double drowning, but it was still not easy saying yes.

After tea she phoned the cardiologist, Dr. Rogan. "I've got to see you while my daughter is here," she said. "It's urgent." She had a touching faith that my brainy assertiveness could succeed where her request had failed. But Dr. Rogan was leaving that day on vacation. He did not have time to meet. She wrung from him a promise to call us back.

At five, the phone rang. My mother asked Dr. Rogan to wait until I could get to the phone in the guest bedroom, but he said he was in a rush. I ran upstairs, knowing that I had perhaps five minutes to talk to a man I'd never met about doing whatever I could to hasten my father's death.

I picked up the receiver and broke in, my voice harsh and tight. I did not thank him for calling, or do any of the things Dale Carnegie suggested I do to win friends and influence people. Instead I blurted out, "I'll cut to the chase." Even if we got a court order, I said, I sensed that he wanted no part in what we had in mind. Dr. Rogan paused and said, "That's right." He'd feel okay about not replacing the pacemaker's battery when it ran down, he said. But turning it off, he said, would be "too active." Later he would tell me that it would have been "like putting a pillow over your father's head."

I put down the phone and walked downstairs, and my mother and I sat on the sofa, held each other, and shook.

My mother handed me a piece of paper the next morning with the number of a hairdresser in the mall below Main Street who cut the hair of the professor in her support group. I took it. Late that afternoon, sporting a nice new chin-length bob, I sat with my mother in the small, brightly lit waiting room of Dr. Fales, their primary care doctor. I'd pulled out my mother's well-organized file holding their "durable power of attorney for health care" documents, and discovered that my father had authorized my mother and me to make his medical decisions when, in the sole opinion of Dr. Fales, he could no longer make his own.

On Dr. Fales's bulletin board was an op-ed piece from the *Hartford Courant* by a fellow internist, fulminating about the low fees Medicare pays for primary care. Dr. Fales ushered us into his office. He had opposed the pacemaker from day one. But turning it off, he said in the fifteen minutes allotted us, was something else again.

"Don't do anything that you would later regret," he said. Without the device, my father might get dizzy or faint, fall, break a hip, and end up in the hospital or a nursing home. "Keep him out of the hospital at all costs," he said. "Try not to call 911." He looked at my mother, and his eyes filled with tears. "Why don't you just let the battery run out?" he said. "It probably only lasts five years, and it's getting close."

Our time was up, and he came around from his desk and gave my mother a hug. When we got home, my mother went into the basement and found a file. The battery of the pacemaker, implanted when my father was seventy-nine, was said to have a ten-year life. We had about five years to go.

When my mother was upset, she meditated or cleaned house. When I was upset, I Googled. That afternoon, I found the 800-number for Compassion and Choices, a successor to the

Hemlock Society, which had first publicly advanced the notion that the fatally ill had a right to die without medical interference and even the right to control the timing of their deaths. Judith Schwarz, a registered nurse in Manhattan with a PhD in nursing, called me back. The law was clear, she said. My father had the right to ask for the withdrawal of *any* medical treatment, even a tiny embedded device like a pacemaker. My mother and I, as his designated health-care proxies, had the right to insist his wishes be followed when he could no longer express them. The cardiologist had an ethical obligation to either deactivate the device or, if he was morally opposed, find us someone who would.

But having legal and moral rights in an era of advanced medical technology, I would learn, was not the same as having practical power. It's easy to say yes to a complex device and devilishly difficult to withdraw that yes. We were at the mercy of a strange new algorithm: those who knew and loved my father best—Dr. Fales, my mother, and I—wanted to let him die naturally but had no power. Those who knew my father least and least understood his suffering were eager to prolong his life and had the know-how and the power to do so.

And so Judith Schwarz recommended I first do everything Dr. Rogan asked for, dotting every *i* and crossing every *t*. I should find a geriatric psychiatrist to declare my father incapable of making his own medical decisions. I should ask Dr. Rogan again to deactivate the device. If he refused, I should insist he find us someone who would. At the same time, I should search independently for a more sympathetic cardiologist. If necessary, we should go to court.

I was not going to get this done in a week.

My every word must be carefully parsed. Following the dicta of St. Thomas Aquinas's Law of Double Effect and centuries of criminal law, I could not say I wanted to hasten my father's death. That could be construed as intent to commit manslaughter. Instead I had to say that my mother and I wanted to "end all mechanical interference with my father's underlying condition." I could not say that we wanted what was best for him. We had to say that "based on our intimate knowledge of his preferences, we were acting exactly as he would if he could speak for himself." We could not say we believed there were fates worse than death. The Supreme Court had affirmed, in the Nancy Cruzan case, that states had an absolute and legitimate interest in the preservation of life. We could not say that my mother was being crushed by caregiving. My mother's suffering had no moral or legal standing. My father, not our family, was the patient.

I should not be rude or threaten a lawsuit. When family members become agitated or disruptive, hospital bioethicists like Katrina Bramstedt may decide that the surrogates lack "decision-making capacity" and the medical team may simply ignore them or go to court and ask to have the troublemakers removed from the job. If that happened, my father's medical proxy wouldn't be worth the paper it was written on.

In a case Bramstedt reported in 2003 in the online *Internal Medicine Journal,* she described a medical guardian who "ranted" and became "agitated and boisterous" in demanding that her relative be allowed to die. She threatened to bring in lawyers, and after her relative developed a hospital-based infection, tried to "fire" the intensive unit team, including Bramstedt, the bioethicist. The patient in question, a sixty-nine-year-old diabetic woman, had been in intensive care for three weeks, on dialysis and on a respirator, after suffering multiple strokes and septic shock (an often fatal bloodstream infection) in the aftermath of her second quadruple bypass surgery. In the ICU, she had picked up another infection from a contaminated line. The woman was apparently too stroke-damaged to communicate and was also suffering from congestive heart failure, a slow and surely fatal condition.

The patient had done everything my parents had been told to do. She'd signed a standard living will asking for the discontinuance of life support if she were comatose or expected to die within six months, In the opinion of the medical team, she was neither. She'd appointed three relatives to act as her medical surrogates when she could not speak for herself. But Bramstedt questioned whether the hostile relative had "decision-making capacity." The request for the removal of life support had been "made in tandem with loud and aggressive behavior," Bramstedt wrote, which "could be a signal that projection is occurring, the emotional fervor being a possible mechanism of expressing the surrogate's own values and preferences," rather than the patient's.

The emotional fervor and aggression of the doctors, and the possibility that they were expressing their own values and preferences, were not discussed in the article. The doctors kept going, and the primary family member withdrew from her role as medical surrogate and said that from then on, she would be a "bystander and a visitor." The second and third relatives deferred to the medical team.

After three more weeks of what Bramstedt called "aggressive treatment" in intensive care, the dying woman was stabilized enough to be sent to a nursing home. Four days later she was brought back to the hospital, feverish, having trouble breathing, and overwhelmed by a second bloodstream infection. This time the medical team did not put her back on life support. She died within hours, according to the hospital's rules, when the medical team decided it was time for her to die, and not a moment before. She had spent most of the final six weeks of her life in intensive care at a cost of hundreds of thousands of dollars—some of it probably paid by Medicare while the rest was absorbed by the hospital and passed on to other patients, indirectly upping health insurance rates—and an uncountable cost in human suffering.

She spent her last weeks, as Sherwin Nuland put it in *How We Die,* among:

> beeping and squealing monitors, the hissings of respirators and pistoned mattresses, the flashing multicolored electronic signals—the whole technological panoply [that] is background for the tactics by which we are deprived of the tranquility we have every right to hope for, and separated from those few who would not let us die alone.

I wanted to spare my father this.

I didn't want him to die because I thought he deserved "death with dignity." I didn't think his dignity was the issue. I didn't want him to die because I judged his "quality of life" to be defective, like a misshapen mail-order sweater that slipped through quality control. I did not think, in the words of the Australian philosopher Peter Singer, that some human lives were "worthy" and others not, and that my father's life was "unworthy" because he was badly damaged. My father was disabled in the eyes of the world before I was born, and I'd felt and expressed more love for him in his helpless dotage than I ever had in his intimidating prime.

I didn't want him to die because my mother and I had dispassionately weighed "the burdens and benefits of continued treatment" as if his life and death were competing brands of refrigerator. We were driven half-mad by love and desperation. I did not want him to die in order to enforce his constitutionally protected right to privacy and autonomy. I did not want him to die because I thought he was useless or because I was ageist. I wanted our family to be held in the loving arms of a larger human community. I wanted doctors to help us. I wanted him to die because I loved him. I wanted to stop our family's suffering. And to do so, Judith Schwarz told me, I would have to speak in a foreign tongue and not as a daughter in grief.

We hadn't created this mess. My father's drawn-out dying and my mother's suffering were the consequence of our culture's idolatrous, one-sided worship of maximum longevity. As far as I was concerned, this violated the way of the universe and was a moral crime. Why were we the ones being judged?

I tried to get my father admitted to a hospice program and learned from a kind nurse on the phone at Middlesex Hospital that my father had "the dwindles": he was sick enough never to get better but not sick enough yet to qualify for Medicare's hospice benefit. She asked if he had an official orange plastic do-not-resuscitate (DNR) bracelet issued by the state of Connecticut. Without it, she said, emergency medical technicians would not honor his paper DNR.

I made another note on my legal pad and again felt like my father's executioner. Only later did I learn that for someone as fragile as my father, a DNR was an almost unequivocal act of mercy. Only 8 percent of people resuscitated outside a hospital leave it alive, and most of them go into nursing homes with too much brain damage to take care of themselves ever again. Only 3 percent of those my father's age recover well enough to return to independent living.

I placed an ad on the local Craigslist offering twenty-five dollars to anyone who would drive to Middletown every weekday evening and spend an hour or so putting my father to bed. My brother Jonathan told me that only an idiot would want such a job. Within days I found a married nursing student who lived in the next town. Relieved, I took a day off, caught the Metro-North commuter train from New Haven to New York City, and proposed some stories to editors. Then I flew back to California.

At home, I found an e-mail waiting from the nursing student: her class schedule had changed and she was turning down the job. I posted another ad on the Hartford Craigslist and from my study in California started calling the motley characters who responded, including several who sounded as if I'd roused them from drug-addled stupors. Finally I found a Chinese-American woman who supported her young daughter by working days in an insurance company office and nights at a Chinese buffet in a distant suburb. I liked her voice. I gave her number to my mother, who liked her too, and three days later, to my relief, Alice Teng quit the buffet and started to work for us.

Thanksgiving and Christmas came and went. I wrote my mother a hectoring letter, telling her it was time to get someone to move in full time. I did not offer to be that person. I searched for a cardiologist willing to turn off the device, and had no luck. In Mill Valley, Brian and I lit fires and held holiday potlucks for his sons and our single friends. I lost five pounds. I dropped out of my book group. I wondered why I wasn't achieving more as a writer.

My mother made another entry in her journal. "This morning he had to be changed from top to bottom including bed-clothes—second time. He slept all morning and even after lunch till three. I then thought we'd go to Wadsworth Park to walk. On the way back he said he'd done a poop—big mess, but managed to clean the car, etc. How I HATE this part." She copied out a haiku by the poet Issa on a three-by-five card and taped it to the bookshelf above her desk: "In this world we walk on the roof of hell, gazing at flowers." On the refrigerator, next to an old pamphlet listing the warning signs of stroke, she stuck a new magnet with a quote paraphrased from Winston Churchill: "When you're going through hell, keep going."

A deepening silence enclosed us.

The only people I felt understood the interior of our lives were Dr. Fales; Teddy, who ran the bustling Middlesex Fruitery on Main Street where my mother and other professors' wives bought their produce; Toni, who still drove up in her battered SUV three days a week; and the bread man at the local Stop & Shop, who each week met my mute father's eyes with a moment of respect and tenderness while taking the loaf of bread my father solemnly handed him to run through the automatic slicer.

I would fly home after each visit to Middletown feeling proud of some small task accomplished and with a knot in my stomach about what was left undone and what might soon need doing. With the exception of Brian, my brothers, and the circle of anonymous women my mother's age whom I met at sporadic Alzheimer's Association support groups, I confided in almost nobody. I would return to my California life expecting no bleed-through. I expected what happened in Connecticut to stay in Connecticut. It was as if it were happening to somebody else's daughter.

I spoke to my friends in shorthand phrases: *Stroke. Pacemaker. Deactivation. Dementia. Mother. Father. Connecticut.* They recoiled. It was easier to say I was furious with Dr. Rogan than to say my heart was breaking. It was easier to talk about medical proxies and a patient's right to medical autonomy and the Nancy Cruzan Supreme Court ruling than about my father's shit-stained dressing gown and my mother's end-of-her-rope violence. Witnessing my parents' suffering was in itself suffering, but by and large I kept the news from myself. I looked around my county for a therapy group for long-distance caregivers like me, and found none. Only with my friend Noelle, whose mother had Alzheimer's, did I say, *For what?* Only to Brian did I say, *My father is dying.* I wrote in my journal that I was "exhausted, resentful, despairing, with nothing left to give."

My mother took my father to Dr. Fales and watched in silence as he attached the state-issued orange plastic DNR bracelet to my father's wrist. Dr. Fales had filled out the forms in triplicate, as you do for a dangerous drug, and ordered the bracelet from a state warehouse. Later that month, my father slipped on the stairs with my mother holding him, tumbling all the way down to the vestibule on top of her, breaking his wrist and turning her black-and-blue from hip to ankle. She debated whether to buy or rent a stair glide, and when Alice said she thought my father had somewhere between six months and a year left of life, decided to rent. A couple of men from a pharmacy supply house in Wethersfield came in a van and installed it. It was another marker of my father's approaching death.

At my prompting, my mother took my father to see Richard Ketai, a geriatric psychiatrist in Middletown. It was another step in my long-term plan, cooked up with the nurse from Compassion and Choices, to validate my mother's legal right to make his medical decisions and get the pacemaker turned off. "Mr. Butler cannot name the year or the month or the season, even though I tell him several times," Dr. Ketai wrote, in a letter declaring my father incapable of understanding, making, or expressing his medical choices. "He can name a watch and a comb but he is utterly unable to name a pen. He denied he had a pacemaker and did not know what one was. It was with some difficulty that he was able to name only two out of his three children."

When I returned to Middletown, it was early spring. A bloom of pale green hovered like mist on the trees outside Dr. Fales's office window. Once again, he sat behind his desk and my mother and I faced him, just as we had not long after my father's first stroke. Again my mother brought up the pacemaker: she'd gotten nowhere. Dr. Rogan said he'd asked around at the Catholic hospital where he had privileges, and no other doctor was any more willing than he. My mother told Dr. Fales that she'd talked to her former internist, the head of Middlesex Memorial Hospital's standing bioethics committee. But because my father was an outpatient, the doctor said, the committee couldn't get involved.

Dr. Fales had warned us earlier that without a pacemaker, my father might get dizzy, fall, and break a hip. But now my father was falling anyway, and Dr. Fales's views had changed. Twice my mother had called 911 when she was too weak to get my father up from the floor alone, and twice she'd had to vehemently resist paramedics who wanted to take him to the emergency room. "You are the one who knows Jeff best, and knows what is best for him," said Dr. Fales. There were tears in his eyes. His own father's Alzheimer's was progressing and he had been hospitalized in Maine. His mother was as exhausted as mine. He was planning to drive north as soon as possible to make sure that the staff at the Maine hospital "kept their hands off" his father and did not resuscitate him. He was a Catholic, Dr. Fales said, but that didn't mean he favored extending life beyond its time.

"Jeff can't communicate," Dr. Fales said to me. "He used to be able to tell me where it hurt. Now he just smiles and agrees with whatever Val and I are saying." He said he'd write us the letter we needed. But as for turning off the pacemaker, he said he didn't know how.

A friend called me from San Francisco. "That's euthanasia," she said flatly and confidently, when I told her what we were trying to do. Brian, who was raised as a Catholic and opposed abortion, said he understood why no cardiologist would help us. "It's the liability," he said. An editor of mine at a mental-health magazine in Washington, DC, gave me the number of a social worker he knew in Baltimore who specialized in aging families. I should take charge, the social worker said over the phone. My father should be moved, against my mother's will if necessary, to a skilled nursing home. I should get my brothers to fly out and help me. That, she seemed to think, was morally preferable to trying to get the pacemaker turned off. "I know what you and your mother want," she said. "But what does your father want?"

The thought made me sick. To which of my fathers did I owe my allegiance? To the semi-intact man who'd come with me on a shuffling walk through Wadsworth Park near the old convent soon after his first stroke, the man who said to me, "But *This! This*"? To the somber man who, a year later, told my mother he was "living too long"? To the beloved and nearly mute man whom I'd promised, "If Val dies, I will take care of you"? To the decrepit eighty-four-year-old who told my mother, "Unfortunately, I come from long-lived people"? To the silent, ancient parrot my father had become? To his brain stem, which would fight to live until the last light in the last cell went out?

Unfortunately, I come from long-lived people.

I could barely articulate our situation to myself; how could I speak in terms my poor father could understand?

It was with some difficulty that he was able to name only two out of his three children.

Would it be anything but cruelty to ask my beloved ruin of a father what he thought about his "quality of life"? To ask him, as Judith Schwarz had suggested, about the kind of funeral he wanted? To ask how he felt about the benefits and burdens of continued treatment?

He denied he had a pacemaker and did not know what one was.

I called a bioethicist at Harvard.

He suggested I imagine that as if by magic, my once-lucid and commanding father could appear at the kitchen table and talk with me for fifteen minutes. I saw my dear father shaking his head in horror over what was no longer a "life" but a slow-motion dying. It didn't help. I sensed that once he died, I would dream of my father and miss his mute, loving smiles. I wanted to melt into the arms of the father I once had and ask him to handle this. I couldn't.

In the course of his eighty-five years, my father had died as a South African schoolboy and been reborn a war hero; he'd died as an able-bodied man and been reborn an amputee, a husband, and a father. He'd died as an Oxford DPhil candidate scraping by on a disabled veteran's pension and been reborn an émigré, an American citizen, and a comfortably retired Wesleyan University professor. I saw no need to sentence him to yet another life, this one stripped of almost every husk of self but a Medicare number and a couple of photographs on a bedside table in the locked "memory care" unit of a nursing home.

I felt in the deepest wells of my being that doing whatever I could to hasten his death (short of manslaughter, for which I had not the courage) was a moral act and a sorrowful necessity. My mother said later, "I can think only of that old-fashioned word, character."

As I groped for a language I could call my own, I thought of Indra's Net, an ancient Buddhist metaphor for the interrelatedness of all life that I'd read about in *The Flower Garland Sutra* one cold, muddy winter in the Plum Village meditation community in southern France. The Net of Indra was a vast, bejeweled matrix spanning and encompassing the whole universe. From every knot hung a jewel, and each jewel reflected the images of all the other jewels hanging from Indra's Net. My father's life was one jewel hanging from a knot in that infinite web, and in that jewel was reflected my life, and my brothers' lives, and my mother's life. Reflected there, too, were the lives of Dr. Fales and Dr. Rogan, all of us infinitely reflecting and affecting one another in a universe without beginning or end, where divine energy flowed from form to form, permeated with light.

In that web, my father's pacemaker and our broken human lives ticked on, not in a universe governed by a god whose rules were written on tablets and interpreted by male priests who'd never spent a day changing adult diapers or listening to the moans of a Nancy Cruzan. They ticked on in a world that could not be reduced to bioethical legalisms, sophistry, evasion, and double-talk.

In the world we lived in, every act and failure to act trailed in their wake widening ripples of suffering. Nowhere I looked did I find Avalokitesvara, the Indian bodhisattva with a hundred eyes and hands who hears the cries of the world and reaches out to help using whatever tool might do the trick. Rarely did I even find the word "suffering" written, much less a map for what to do when the ones you love are drowning in it.

Two women rang my parents' doorbell and introduced themselves. One was an occupational therapist and the other a visiting nurse. Unbeknownst to us, Dr. Fales, alarmed by my father's frequent falls, had referred us to a program I'd never heard of called palliative care. I would later learn that it is a growing, relatively new medical specialty that emphasizes relieving physical and emotional pain. It represents a ray of hope in our broken medical system. Palliative care, the nurse explained, offered home visits, a coordinated medical team, and a social worker. Unlike hospice, it did not require a medical finding that my father would die within six months. The emphasis would be on caring—for all of us—rather than trying to cure my incurable father. The nurse gave my mother the phone number of a "lift and assist" service at the fire department, an alternative to 911, to help her get my father up without facing a push to take him to the emergency room. The occupational therapist walked through the house and pointed out small rugs that could be taken up to lessen the chances of my father falling. She suggested my mother buy a commode and a baby monitor for my father's bedroom.

Finally we were not alone.

At dinner I saw my father examine the plastic DNR bracelet on his wrist, trying to read its blurred words with slow, parrot-like curiosity. Nobody, I sensed, had talked to him about it. What would we say?

As my parents and I finished watching the news together, the doorbell rang, Alice Teng walked in, and my father brightened. He rose unsteadily to roll the television back to its accustomed nook, but my mother sharply said no: he'd recently tipped it over. "You show me how, Jeff," Alice said gracefully, and he obediently hovered behind her as she rolled it away. He followed her to the stair glide, where she helped him sit down, showed him again where to put his feet, buckled him in, and pressed the button gliding him upward. I did not believe in angels, but I thanked whatever powers there might be for Alice. Jesus said that the stone the builders rejected would become the cornerstone. Alice treated my father with dignity and saved my mother from herself and her exhaustion, leaving the house each night, after cleaning his teeth and putting him to bed, with a cheery, "Good night, Jeff!" She and Toni were our cornerstones. It didn't matter that they were paid for the mercy they showed us. I felt an almost religious gratitude to Toni and Alice, who gave their hearts, wisdom, and gentleness to us, near-strangers.

The situation was better, but my mother was worse. She could not sleep. In the mornings, when I tried to talk about hiring someone to move in, she felt faint. She put her head between her legs at the kitchen table. She went to the living room and lay down on the sofa.

*   *   *

I joined my mother in her yoga routine one morning as my father slept. As we stretched our backs up and down in cat-and-cow, she told me, for the third time since my plane landed, that I looked anorexic. Again I felt my heart sink and again I asked her to drop it. Would I never be okay in her eyes—not too thin or too fat, too close or too distant, too bossy or too meek, too needy or too independent, too sloppily dressed or wearing too many colors? "Katy," she said, "You have no sense of humor!"

When we were done, I went upstairs, changed out of my yoga clothes, and quietly called Southwest to move my reservation a day closer. I was not going to criticize, condemn, or complain. I knew that the only way to win an argument with my mother was to avoid one. When she started needling me like this, I told myself, it was her way of saying it was time I went home.

I took my father for a last walk later that morning, the two of us heading down the margin of the busy road to the old Cenacle convent. We planned to walk to a stop sign a long block from the house. His wheezing was so loud that it frightened me. When I suggested turning back, he spat out, between labored breaths, with the old contempt I remembered well from our warring years, "You're . . . the One . . . that's *Scared*," and marched doggedly on. The stroke-damaged man who had walked by himself to the Wesleyan pool three times a week was a superhero compared with the angry shut-in old body now shuffling beside me.

At lunch, my mother took my hand. "I don't want you to leave," she said, and she began to weep. "I want you to stay longer." I looked into her blue eyes, swimming with tears, and held her hand: she was raw, open, loving, honest, and beautiful. I didn't say, *I can't bear your calling me anorexic*. I didn't say, *Stop and I'll stay*. I stroked her hand and made comforting noises, but I made no move to change my flight.

The morning I was set to go home to San Francisco, I hesitated at my father's door, and then went in and woke him. It was 6:30, and the sky was dark outside the window. He opened his eyes and smiled at me. "Toni's taking me to the airport," I said, not sure if he would understand.

"Should I get up? Am I coming?" he said.

"No," I said, and kissed him on the cheek. "Good-bye," I said. "Go back to sleep. I love you."

Three weeks later, my mother called me in California and said, "Come."

V

ACCEPTANCE

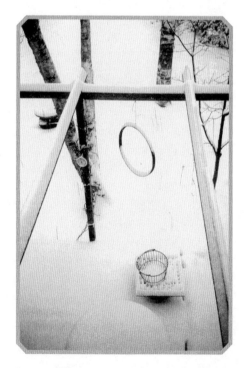

Winter at Pine Street, Middletown, Connecticut.

CHAPTER 14

THE ART OF DYING

My father's bronchitis had worsened. My mother had not called a doctor. In the daytime, he slept. At night he thrashed around in their old master bedroom, sometimes getting up and falling, as my mother, drained of sleep, listened via the baby monitor from the guest bedroom and came in to get him back into bed. His breathing grew worse, his mind more agitated. The palliative-care nurse came one morning and put her ear on his gurgling chest. He had pneumonia, she said. He was finally dying decisively enough to qualify for hospice. Thanks to our involvement with her program, he would not meet his death in intensive care after a panicked stop in an emergency room. The nurse called the hospital and made the arrangements, and my mother called an ambulance. He was taken to Middlesex Hospital's inpatient hospice unit, fighting as if for his life, kicking and biting and telling the orderlies to "bugger off." Toni visited. She asked him if he knew who she was, and he opened one eye and fixed her with a baleful and knowing look. He ate a full dinner, and then was shot full of morphine.

By the time I got there, he was lying silently in bed, his lungs slowly filling with fluid, unreachable, his eyes shut, breathing as hard and regularly as a machine.

The hospice unit was homey and peaceful. Pamphlets told us that my father's hearing would be the last sense to go. They suggested we read aloud to him, play his favorite music, and say whatever in our hearts was left unsaid. At the end of the hall was a carpeted living room with a phone and a comfortable couch and videotapes for the families. There was a nondenominational chapel about twice the size of a walk-in closet, a kitchen, a coffee machine, and a refrigerator full of sheet cake.

My mother knelt by his bed, holding his hand and stroking his hair, weeping and begging for forgiveness for her impatience. The beginnings of a tear oozed out from under my father's eyelid, and a nurse said to my mother, *Stop. You're making him cry.* I was again ambushed by their love and my continuing failure to understand it.

My mother sat by him in agony. She beseeched the doctors and nurses to increase his morphine dose and end his suffering. She kept asking about turning off the pacemaker. By the time the hospice unit called Dr. Rogan's cardiology practice it was a Saturday, and the doctor on call refused to authorize deactivation. Apparently no message was given to Dr. Rogan, who later told me that he'd have turned it off if he'd known. A month after my father's death, a joint committee of the American Heart Association, the Heart Rhythm Society, and the American College of Cardiology would issue a "consensus statement" declaring that it was morally and legally acceptable to deactivate a pacemaker if the patient wished, and that it was neither assisted suicide nor euthanasia. That would come, of course, too late for us.

And so followed five days of hard labor.

Love can look heartless. We did not give my father oxygen or food or an IV of saline or a cup of water. If we had, we would have only slowed the shutting down of his organs and the drawn-out process of his death. A nurse told us that dying from not eating or drinking is not painful, and I myself had fasted for days without distress, but I could not forget the gospel of Matthew, in which Jesus says, "For I was hungry, and you gave me meat; I was thirsty, and you gave me drink." Never before in history have so many sons, daughters, and spouses been forced to treat those they love like this at the end.

We would not treat a dog this way.

When death takes just a few days, it is easy, or at least possible, to hold the dying person in the center of your attention. When you have already attended a slowly dying person for years, it's harder. I could barely bear to be there and listen to his labored breathing and my mother's weeping. I left my mother with him and went to Pelton's drugstore on Main Street and bought a copy of *Elle* magazine. I came back to the hospital and waited for my brothers to come and for my father to die. I went shopping for shoes at Marshalls, once with my mother and once alone. I came back in my new shoes and sat by his bed and read *Elle* and held his hand. I was fifty-nine and had never before sat at a deathbed.

Once upon a time we knew how to die. We knew how to sit at a deathbed. We knew how to die and how to sit because we saw people we loved die all through infancy, childhood, youth, middle age, and old age: deaths we could not make painless, deaths no machine could postpone. The deaths of our ancestors were not pretty. Some died roaring in pain. But through the centuries we tutored ourselves in the art of dying by handing down stories about how those we loved met their deaths.

*   *   *

When St. Francis was in his forties in 1226, having suffered years of illness and sensing his death was near, he "caused himself to be stripped of all his clothing, and to be laid upon the ground, that he might die in the arms of the Lady Poverty." Death did not come as quickly as he expected. He was taken back into the house where he'd lain and lifted back to his bed. He asked his monks to sing him his own "Canticle of the Sun." "Praised be my Lord for our sister the moon, and for the stars, which He has set clear and lovely in heaven," the monks sang, and they added new lines that St. Francis had recently written: "Praised be my Lord for our sister the death of the body, from whom no man escapeth." The next day, "when his pains were some little abated," St. Francis put his hand on the head of each of his monks, and gave his blessing "unto all the Order present, absent, and to come, even unto the world's end.

"Then as the sun was setting, there was a great silence," went one version of St. Francis's death story, as recounted by a Victorian essayist:

> As the brethren were gazing on his face, desiring to see some sign that he was still with them, behold a great multitude of birds came about the house wherein he lay, and flying a little way off did make a circle round the roof, and by their sweet singing did seem to be praising the Lord with him.

Such holy deaths were not reserved for saints. In the fifteenth century, when Europe was so decimated by the Black Death that there weren't enough Catholic priests around to give Last Rites, our ancestors created road maps for the deathbed. The earliest Latin versions, written by priests, were called, simply, *Ars moriendi*, or *The Art of Dying*. The English versions, revised over time to fit Protestant theology, included *The Boke of Crafte of Dyinge*, *The Art and Craft to Know Well to Die*, and *Rules and Exercises of Holy Dying*.

The *Ars moriendi* did not sugarcoat the death agony, and they described scenes foreign to us now. Relatives and friends gathered at the bedside at home and followed the script of the *Ars moriendi*, asking the right questions and saying the prescribed prayers, giving the dying person reassurance and hope. The hallmark of a good death was not an absence of suffering but the ability to meet it with faith, courage, and acceptance. Stoicism was not required: in 1651, the Anglican theologian Jeremy Taylor wrote in his *Rules and Exercises of Holy Dying* that it was okay to groan on the deathbed.

The *Ars moriendi* did not pretend that dying was the pinnacle of a lifetime of meaningful growth experiences. Their authors lamented, even in 1491, that "men seek sooner and busier after medicine for the body than for the soul." They portrayed the deathbed not as a lowly place of helplessness and meaningless suffering but as a mighty, transcendent battleground where angels and demons struggled for control of the soul. The dying person, not the doctor, was the star of the show. Her anguish was framed as a series of temptations to sin: wavering faith, despair, impatience, regret for past misdeeds, reluctance to say good-bye, and especially fear of death and hell. Dying was not merely a physical agony; it was also a spiritual ordeal. Its suffering had meaning. The brave person did not battle Death but regarded dying as a test of one's trust in God, an earthly purification to be followed by a heavenly reward, a sacred rite of passage as profound and familial as a christening or a wedding. The Good Death was marked by last words, treasured by the survivors, expressing repentance for past misdeeds, acceptance of God's will, and confidence in his mercy.

My father did not die that way. He did not say three times,

as the *Boke of the Crafte of Dyinge* recommended, "Into thine hands, Lord, I commit my soul." I did not ask him, as I would later learn that the *Ars moriendi* recommended, if he asked for God's forgiveness, if he forgave those who'd harmed him, if he forsook all the goods of the world, and if he thanked God for Christ's sacrifice. I held his hand and said almost nothing.

All I could see was his closed eyes and his labored breathing.

Dr. Elisabeth Kübler-Ross, in her 1969 bestseller, theorized that dying people moved through stages of denial, anger, bargaining, depression, and acceptance, though not necessarily in that order. If anything, my father had moved backward over time, from acceptance to depression and anger.

He was doing the long, hard work of his dying in a small, windowless interior room within his own body, his once-booming and argumentative voice stopped by dementia, deafness, stroke and brain damage, pneumonia and morphine. If he cried out inside that small interior room, if he yearned for reconciliation with his estranged son Michael, if he desired Jonathan's forgiveness for having been a neglectful father, if he forgave my mother, if he saw white light or his dead brother Guy welcoming him to paradise, I will never know.

The well-known hospice and palliative-care doctor Ira Byock counsels the dying and those they love to say to each other some version of these words: *I love you. Thank you. Please forgive me. I forgive you. Good-bye.* My father and I said none of those things.

My father just breathed, a terrible loud, ever-louder breathing, like someone working very hard at something, like someone building a wall, like someone delivering a baby. As he breathed day and night, as his lungs filled with fluid, he was washed and changed and kept clean by kind paid strangers, and my mother cried and pled for forgiveness, and I came and went and held his hand. There was nothing left for us to do. In wordless ways, over seven years, I had already said, *I love you. Thank you. Please forgive me. I forgive you.* I comforted myself with the memory of waking him on the last morning of my last trip home, when I'd said, "Good-bye. Go back to sleep. I love you."

As my mother and I made our passages to and fro through the quiet streets of Middletown, we looked like anyone else there, shopping for a roasted chicken or opening a car window or just walking dully along. In the evenings at Pine Street, we found messages from some of my father's old colleagues on the answering machine—the outward and visible sign of a community that still loved him and had wanted to connect throughout his long illness but often had not known how. My mother, in her agony and shame, or in her émigré self-reliance, or in her reflexive drawing-in to her core, discouraged them from coming to the hospital. He was unconscious, she said. What was the point?

No all-night lighted square of window signaled to our neighbors, who could not see my parents' carefully sited house from the street in any case, that our ancient vigil was underway. My two brothers were still on the West Coast, throwing clothes into their suitcases and shopping for funeral clothes. I dreaded their arrival. Brian pleaded with me to let him fly in and support me, but I still had not learned how to say, "I need you," and I said no.

My father was a guest in a hotel for the dying. The hospice nurses, practiced at filling the spiritual vacuums of contemporary life, would minister to us unobtrusively, the way priests and family members once did. I was grateful. One calm nurse explained to me that nobody could say exactly when my father's death would come, but that it *would* come: thus she gently disabused me of my fantasy that maybe my father would get better somehow and come home. To the hospice nurse, death was not an emergency. It was part of the plan. She told me that as the time got closer, my father's feet and hands would turn blue, and her map of the coming of death calmed me.

She told me that thanks to the morphine, my father wasn't suffering, but I didn't believe her. I knew that if we gave the word he'd be gurneyed immediately to intensive care, where he'd be shot full of antibiotics and hooked up to intravenous lines and perhaps a respirator, and perhaps survive to die another day. I wanted my father to die as quickly as possible. I wanted him not to die until my brothers got there. I felt as if we were killing him. I did not want him to die at all.

I had prayed for his death, awaited his death, and expected his death. And now that it was nearly here, I was surprised it had come.

My ancestors often did not know what they were dying *of*, but knew when they were dying. Sometimes they saw their deaths coming, and comforted those they loved ahead of time. When hope was pointless, they fell back on the ancient technology of acceptance. "I do want you not to fret about me," my Quaker great-grandfather James wrote in 1876 to his mother, Mary Watts Butler, from the farm where he was staying in the English countryside, stricken by the tuberculosis that a generation earlier had deformed his father's backbone and killed his grandfather and his aunt. James was only in his early twenties when he wrote, "We all know even if we don't often think about it that we all must pass away & that our happy family circle must inevitably gradually dissolve." His younger sister Mary had died suddenly of typhoid, at the age of thirteen, in a Quaker boarding school, and her death, he wrote, "spoke forcibly to all of us. It told us of the uncertainty of life & of the necessity of preparing for death. I trust that I may join my dear sister, & that as we all one by one quit this earth we may one by one re-form the family circle in Heaven." James's doctors could do nothing for his health beyond suggesting that he move to a sunny climate. Soon after he wrote his mother the letter, he sailed for South Africa, settled in the desert, and to everyone's surprise, recovered enough to start the *Midland News and Karoo Farmer,* marry a farm girl named Lettie Collett, and sire seven healthy sons and daughters, all of whom lived long lives.

At my father's bedside, I drew no comfort from the notion that our family circle would ever be reconstituted in heaven and even less from the notion, held by some of my fellow Buddhists, that my father would be reborn in another form. I believed that rebirth and heaven were myths, comforting stories for children afraid of the dark. I believed that my father existed only as long as the material conditions supporting his life existed, and that when those conditions disappeared, he would disappear too, leaving behind only memory traces in our minds, like a trail of bubbles in a cloud chamber. The molecules of his body would become part of cells in other bodies: plants, lizards, vinca minor, figs. His love for me would live on inside me, just as my brother Jonathan's sense of abandonment would live on inside him. That was the limit of my belief in eternal life.

All I could see were his closed eyes and his labored breathing. The pacemaker kept delivering its tiny pulses.

His breathing grew ragged and his feet, as the nurse had warned me, slowly started to turn blue. Sometimes yellow phlegm dribbled out of his mouth onto the cloth the nurses had placed by his pillow. In the presence of his extreme helplessness and suffering, I sometimes felt horror and disgust. But I had no prayers to say.

I left my mother and went alone to the Wesleyan library, where I looked up citations and drafted a letter to the Middlesex

Hospital bioethics committee, pleading to get the pacemaker deactivated. At four in the afternoon, I abandoned my draft, shut down the computer, and surrendered. I would stop shooting myself with the Second Arrow. I would accept the things I could not change. I could not shorten my father's suffering or hasten his death. I would stop being a warrior and a medical guardian and simply be a grieving daughter.

I drove back to the hospital. My mother was gone. I held my father's warm hand and felt his strong pulse, his energy still flowing. He was still my father and I was still his daughter. I held his hand for hours, letting him give his love to me one last time.

In a study of Zen funeral rituals in Japan, William Bodiford, an anthropologist, stated that, "One of the purposes of religion is to guide the living through the experience of death." My mother and I craved the sacred, but we did not know how to bring it to my father's deathbed. We'd attended Buddhist retreats and read Pema Chödrön and meditated alone, but neither one of us had embedded ourselves in a local Buddhist *sangha,* or community. And only through the flesh and blood of other imperfect human beings could religion have guided us through my father's death. I asked a hospice nurse for a Buddhist chaplain, but in Middletown, where most of the residents are African-American Protestants or Polish-American, Latin-American, and Sicilian-American Catholics, she knew of none.

A gentle woman in a blue dress introduced herself: she was Elizabeth Miel, a volunteer Episcopalian chaplain. We sat together, one on each side of my father's bed. I told her that my father's mother had been Anglican, and that when I was a little girl in Oxford, my parents had gone to communion regularly, and I, to the Sunday school at St. Michael and All Angels.

There I was told that God was everywhere and saw every-

thing, and I imagined God as a series of transparent shower cur-
tains embedded with multitudinous fish eyes, moving in every
wind. At night I'd kneel by my bed and beg for a sign of His reality. But God was silent, at least in the forms that I expected him
to speak. Until Saturday, when I would ride my bike to green
fields bordering a stream and lie heart-side down in the mossy
grass, letting the green energy rise up into me. There, I had an
inkling of a wholeness beyond the logic of my family. I didn't
have to work for it. All I had to do was put myself in a position
to receive. Green things continued to feed what I called my soul
long after I abandoned any hope of ever seeing the luminous
fish eyes of God waving in the transparent wind. I worshipped
holy water and holy dirt long before I called it prayer.

There was nothing green in the hospital room.

The chaplain offered to give my father Last Rites. I looked over
my shoulder, worried that my mother might walk in. I said yes.

The chaplain opened a little stainless-steel canister containing cotton batting soaked with olive oil, and made the sign of the
cross on my father's forehead with her thumb. Opening her Book
of Common Prayer, she began reading from the Litany at the Time
of Death. "Look on this your servant Jeffrey lying in great weakness and comfort him with promise of life everlasting," she read.

My shoulders let down. I didn't think my father would mind.
It might comfort him. It was comforting me.

"Set him free from every bond, that he may rest with all your
saints in the eternal habitations where with the Father and the
Holy Spirit you live and reign." I liked the notion that the soul
of my poor laboring father was going *somewhere,* even into the
glorious company of the saints in whom I did not believe. "May
his soul rest in peace," the chaplain said.

She handed me a little blue brochure with a drawing of
someone with a halo on the cover, and together she and I read
aloud the Twenty-Third Psalm, which would comfort me on

many nights to come, when I could not sleep. "Yea, though I walk through the valley of the shadow of death, I will fear no evil," we said together. I barely knew the chaplain's name. I let a breath fill the hole in my aching heart, and the warmth spread outward. "Thou anointest my head with oil. Surely goodness and mercy shall follow me all the days of my life, and I will dwell in the house of the Lord forever."

After a little while, Elizabeth got up and closed the door behind her.

My brother Jonathan arrived, touched my father's shoulder, and said, "It's all good."

Three times in the course of my father's long life, he had taken a step toward the ferryboat across the dark river, only to be blocked by luck, or fate, or medicine. First came his brush with accidental death as a teenager in the 1930s, on the warm desert night when he failed to catch up with the red taillights of the stolen car that bore two of his closest friends to their deaths in a ditch in the veld outside Cradock. Then came battlefield death, from whose strong arms doctors wielding penicillin and surgical knives wrested him in 1944 in a field hospital in Italy. Then came his natural death, curling like a cat in his slowing heart and stalking away when the pacemaker went in. Then came all the tiny deaths suffered as he lost, neuron by neuron, his memory, freedom, sight, hearing, balance, and personality. Now, at last, his final, merciful, difficult, and belated death threaded its way through every man-made obstacle, flying in on leather wings through an upstairs window quietly opened by my mother, who, by refusing to give my father water, food, or antibiotics, fulfilled her marriage's final, tender, and brutal vow.

With my mother alone at his side the next afternoon, my father's lungs and brain gave out, and he stopped breathing.

*   *   *

I got her phone call at the house and cried out like an animal. He had died without me. Then I realized he was no longer suffering and that he had not been alone—she'd been with him. As Jonathan and I headed for the hospital, our brother Michael was on the outskirts of Bradley Airport outside Hartford, hastily signing the papers to pick up his rental car. A hospice nurse hung a blue light on the outside of my father's door.

Inside my father's chest, the pacemaker was sending its tiny pulses to dead muscle.

We sat in silence, the three of us. We read no poems and said no prayers. My cell phone rang, and like a fool, I flipped it open and talked to a man from a cremation service. I did not know enough to make the moment sacred, and I was bereft of forms that could have told me what to do or say.

We did not stay long enough to see peace descend on his features, although my brother Michael said that when he went alone to the hospital room a few hours later, he saw translucence and beauty in our father's face, a reflection perhaps of the bliss of letting go and stopping all forms of striving.

CHAPTER 15

AFTERWARD

When my great-grandfather James was sixty-seven, four decades after his nearly fatal brush with tuberculosis, he knew he was not long for this world. Increasingly listless and white, he grew short of breath while climbing the stairs at his newspaper office in the South African desert. The trouble was his heart. His doctor recommended he rest from running the newspaper and sip a daily tot of whiskey, which was out of the question because James was a strict Quaker and a teetotaler. The doctor could offer little more: it was 1923, and heart surgery and most heart medications did not yet exist. After a holiday on a relative's sheep farm did little to restore him, James wrote to his English relatives that he was planning to turn over the newspaper to my grandfather, his son Ernest.

One winter afternoon, James walked unsteadily down Bree

Street to the Cradock Methodist church, and as he'd promised, gave a talk promoting temperance to its Young Men's Guild. According to letters his unmarried younger sister Eliza Butler later wrote to their English relatives—letters I later found in a file in a South African library—James spoke sitting down. When he finished, a young man asked a question. My great-grandfather said, "I think we have come to the end," slumped forward, lost consciousness, and died.

Nobody knew whether he'd had a stroke or suffered a cardiac arrest or a heart attack. Nobody attempted to revive him: CPR was forty years away. Dying, death, and mourning were all of a piece then. His body was brought straight home in the town ambulance. Family letters make no mention of any involvement by a funeral home, and it's probable that his body was simply washed and prepared for burial in the ancient way, not by strangers but by members of the family or household servants. His daughter Mary and my grandmother Alice made wreaths and arranged bouquets to decorate the drawing room, and there his open coffin was placed, with a handkerchief over his face to keep flies away. Relatives and townspeople visited. "I stole in, and Mary followed me," wrote his sister Eliza to her siblings in London. "She uncovered his face, and there he was, so calm and peaceful, pale and stiff, eyes closed, surely at rest. I said, 'Poor old Jimmy . . . ' and the tears flowed freely." Nobody expected her to move to "closure" within six months. Before the public funeral at the Methodist church, Eliza, Mary, and the rest of the town's few Quakers held a silent meeting. The coffin was taken by horse-drawn carriage to the church and then to the graveyard, with almost everyone in Cradock, including many people of color, walking behind it. One man's death was still the business, then, of everyone in town. The bell from the church steeple—one of the tallest buildings in Cradock—tolled over the town and into the desert.

The tolling of a bell to announce a death was a ritual stretching back to the Middle Ages, and it kept the reality of death in everyone's mind. "It was a sad noise to hear our bell to toll and ring so often to-day, either for deaths or burials; I think five or six times," wrote Samuel Pepys in his diary on July 30, 1665, during the Great Plague of London. "In the City died this week 7,496 and of them 6,102 of the plague. But it is feared that the true number of the dead, this week is near 10,000; partly from the poor that cannot be taken notice of, through the greatness of the number, and partly from the Quakers and others that will not have any bell ring for them."

The news of my father's death was posted on the Wesleyan Web site.

When we got home from the hospital, my mother did not weep. She walked through the door at Pine Street, took off her jacket, picked up my father's sheepskin mitten from its home on the shelf above the coat pegs, walked out to the garage, and flung it into the garbage can. She called Pelton's Medical Supply Company in Wethersfield, owner of the stair glide. "Take it out as soon as you can," she said. "I can't bear to look at it."

Dying is hard on the dying. Death is hard on the living.

She went to the living room and took the waterproof cushion off the wrought-iron outdoor chair my father had used when he could no longer raise himself from the couch. She put the chair back on the deck. She undid the safety pins from the stretchy black strip of ribbon that had turned my father's blue-and-white checked dinner napkin into the most elegant possible bib. In the master bedroom, she stripped the waterproof plastic cover from my father's mattress. She threw out the long-handled comb I'd found for him in a disability catalog.

There was a thud. A small brown bird had flown into the

glass wall of the vestibule and broken its neck. It lay still in the low leaves of the vinca minor. My mother opened the front door, picked up the bird by its feet, and flung it violently down the slope, deep into the woods. She came back in, slammed the door, and cried out, "Jeff! I told you not to die before me!"

I had never understood the deeps of my parents' marriage, below its glittering and bickering surface—how glamorous they looked as a couple, their parties, their trips to Maine and to watch horsemen race the Palio in Siena, their in-jokes, her carping and bossiness, his occasional outbursts of "you bloody harridan!" and his withdrawal, year after year, to work in his downstairs study. I thought that whatever remained of their love had burned away, leaving behind only duty, exhaustion, anger, fear, and dependence.

In my father's army-green file cabinets downstairs, which once held notes about alfalfa crop yields in Cradock in the 1920s, I would find after my mother's death the remorseful and tender love letters he'd written her while on a research trip to Africa in his midsixties, after he'd taken her for granted once too often and she threatened to leave him. I'd never written anyone such letters, and hadn't treasured the ones Brian had written to me. In her desk I would find notes my father had written her before his stroke and she lovingly collected, each signed with a smiling face in a top hat or a striped jersey. I would remember him watching her comb her long, wet gray hair in the kitchen sunlight sometime in the 1980s and his saying to me, "Isn't she beautiful?" when all I could see was a woman of sixty, a woman as old as I was soon to be. I would find the birthday letters he'd eked out to her when he could barely remember the date.

I had been deaf to the chords and rhythms of their love. I'd never loved anyone the way they loved each other. I had kept Brian at arm's length for seven years. I was starting to understand how much I did not understand.

My heart ached as I silently watched my mother rocket through the house, plundering and sacking. I went to the garage and pulled my father's mitten from the garbage can where she'd flung it. I wanted to touch something intimate of my father's before she chucked it all. The mitten was covered with kitchen rot and already permeated with stink. "You've got it bad," said my brother Jonathan, making a face. He said he'd made peace long ago with our father's neglect and had given his resentments to God. He was grateful he'd arrived soon enough to say good-bye but not so soon that he'd had to sit around with us being miserable. I put the stinking mitten back in the garbage and went upstairs to my father's bathroom, where I found the waterproof black plastic Timex, dusted with dandruff, that I'd bought him to water-walk at the Wesleyan pool. I put it in my pocket.

By nightfall, my mother had erased from the house almost every visible sign of my father's six and a half years of illness. All that remained was the lowered hook in the entryway, with two spackled holes above it where the original hook had hung.

My mother had never forgotten Jessica Mitford's 1963 best-seller *The American Way of Death,* which both investigated and mocked the American funeral industry. She did not even want to give the funeral director a set of clothes to burn my father's body in. "Naked we shall return," she told him, as we sat around the dining-room table going over the cremation contract. Only after my brother Michael asked her to consider whether she really wanted to watch her husband's corpse plunge into the flames in a clear plastic bag did she relent and allow me to hand over a blue cotton shirt I'd once given my father as a Christmas present, and a pair of his frayed khakis. She signed the papers, asked the undertaker about a ring he was wearing, wrote the check, shut the door behind him, and told my brothers and me that she wanted no memorial service. Phony eulogies made her skin crawl.

"The dead don't care," she said, quoting the undertaker and essayist Thomas Lynch.

But the living do, I said.

The funeral home arranged to have my father's body transported from the hospital morgue to the Swan Funeral Home in Old Saybrook on Long Island Sound. We would not wash and dress it ourselves, the way my great-grandfather's relatives did. The funeral home had several cremations ahead of ours. My father's body lay refrigerated somewhere while my brothers and I planned the memorial service.

We did not call it a "celebration of life." We were mourning a death, and we knew it. We did not hire a minister to say vague things about a man he did not know. I downloaded a do-it-yourself memorial template and my brothers and I patched something postmodern together, the way people do now, out of poetry and music we liked, and the tradition of public sharing borrowed from Quaker and 12-step meetings. While my father's body lay refrigerated at the crematory, we played a CD of *shakuhachi* flute, and two hundred people, most of them old friends connected with Wesleyan, filed into the university's brownstone chapel.

Toni, our caregiver, sat with the family in the front row, Alice Teng by choice with her daughter, quietly in back. My brother Michael, the actor who'd inherited my mother's elegance, presided in black turtleneck and black jeans. He read from Dietrich Bonhoeffer and invited people to come one by one up to the lectern, where they remembered, as people do, our father's best qualities and their love for him.

One faculty wife, a devout Christian, said her young son had asked her whether my father would be reunited with his lost arm in heaven. Toni said that "Mr. Butler" was smiling down at us and no longer suffering. Ben Carton, the handsome former student who'd been close to a surrogate son and visited my parents often, remembered being up on our roof with my father helping him make a repair, and listening to him describe how he watched his footprints fill up with blood after he was wounded in Italy. In all his heroic telling and retelling of this tale, my father never told me, as he had Ben, that he watched the volume of his gushing blood and estimated how many minutes he had left to live.

My brother Jonathan stood up last, in a dark shirt, a wide tie, and a pale seersucker suit he'd bought the day before at Syms on our mother's credit card. He said he was "the black sheep of the family"—the one who'd never gone to college and who drove trucks for a living. He remembered helping my father build the living-room bookshelves in the basement wood shop at Pine Street when he was a boy, using old carpentry tools—forged at the turn of the century, it happened, in nearby Meriden—that my father had inherited from *his* father Ernest, and that Jonathan now used in his California wood shop.

Jonathan read out the Rudyard Kipling poem "If." The chapel filled with the ghostly whistling of "Colonel Bogey's March," the signature tune of the British POWs in a movie my father loved, *The Bridge on the River Kwai.* At the close, I read a Shakespearean funeral poem, a perfect hymn for nonbelievers, its rhythms majestic, its promises minimal, its comforts true and plain:

> Fear no more the heat o' the sun
> Nor the furious winter's rages
> Thou thy worldly task hast done
> Home art gone, and ta'en thy wages.
> Golden lads and girls all must,
> As chimney-sweepers, come to dust.

A hired Wesleyan music professor stood up in the balcony, raised her trumpet, and played taps. Alice, the evening caregiver who seemed like an angel to me, left a bunch of white flowers in the chapel, with a note echoing her nightly leave-taking: "Good night, Jeff."

After the funeral home dropped off my father's ashes, I carried the brown plastic box into the woods of the old Cenacle convent, where soon after the stroke, I'd asked him if his life was still worth living and where, six years later, I'd taken him into a copse and bounced a turd out of his underwear. It was late April, still overcast and cold.

"How fleeting is a lifetime! Who in this world today can maintain a human form for even a hundred years? There is no knowing whether I will die first or others, whether death will occur today or tomorrow," reads "White Ashes," by the fifteenth century Japanese priest Rennyo, often read at American funerals held by the Jodo Shinshu branch of Buddhism.

> We depart one after another more quickly than the dewdrops on the roots or the tips of the blades of grasses. So it is said. Hence, we may have radiant faces in the morning, but by evening we may turn into white ashes. Once the winds of impermanence have blown, our eyes are instantly closed and our breath stops forever. Then, our radiant face changes its color, and the attractive countenance like peach and plum blossoms is lost.

"What is left after the body has been cremated and has turned into the midnight smoke is just white ashes," said Rennyo. "Words cannot describe the sadness of it all."

By the side of the stream, I opened the box, scooped a handful of ashes out of the plastic bag, and threw them into the swirling water, watching the heavier pieces of his bones sink and the dust float downstream, a chalky veil on the skin of the water.

There were some curious spiraled metal wires, perhaps the leads that once ran from his pacemaker to his heart, among the white ashes and pieces of bone.

My father had wanted his body to be buried in Indian Hill Cemetery, on the western fringe of the Wesleyan campus. Decades before his stroke, he'd shown me exactly where he wanted his headstone placed: on the low brow of a hill, facing across Vine Street toward the Wesleyan freshman dining hall and a small colonial cemetery known as West Burying Ground. It was a family tradition to wander through Indian Hill, the last redoubt of the Wapanoags, reading the eighteenth- and nineteenth-century headstones and noting the Polish, English, and Irish names listed along with their places of birth: Cork, Bristol, Donegal. The Sicilian-Americans, who'd mostly arrived later, were buried in the newer Catholic cemetery on the other side of High Street.

No trip home was complete without a visit with my father to Indian Hill's Civil War memorial—a low stone enclosure on a slope overlooking the old Route 66. A boy-man in a gray granite uniform and billed cap stood watch above a score of small stubby markers bearing the names of the dead. My father loved it as a historian and as a veteran. He, too, wanted to leave a headstone with his particulars, so that in the future people could piece together something of the history of Middletown and its successive waves of immigration.

But my mother was set on cremation, she had earned the right to decide a hundred times over, the dead don't care, and in any case, there would soon be no more Butlers left to visit a grave in Middletown. After my brother Jonathan caught his plane, I went up to Indian Hill with my mother and Michael to bury some of my father's ashes there.

We walked to the crown of the hill. It was sunny and warm, close to midday. I'd brought a trowel and a plastic ziplock bag of his ashes. My mother sat down on the ground and, for the first time since my father's death, began to weep. She spoke to him as if he were alive and fully functioning, as though they were alone together, intimate, man and wife.

I grabbed the trowel and cut into the earth. She cried out, "Oh Katy! Don't stab it like that!" She took the trowel from me, and tenderly lifted out the clods as if the earth and the grass were living things. Still weeping and talking to my father, she took a few ashes out of the plastic Baggie and put them into the ground. Then she put the clods back and made a circle of daisies around them.

She stood up, sobbing loudly. She wanted to go home at once. I didn't. I wanted to scatter more ashes at the Civil War monument and take comfort in the thought of my father there, among his soldiers. Full of rage and grief, I broke away and sat down beneath a tree near the monument and put my head on my knees and wept. There my brother Michael found me and gently took me back to the car. I was still Katy and my mother was still Valerie. We had transcended nothing. I would need her forgiveness, as she would need mine, until the end of our days.

I had expected that my father's death would catapult my mother and me into a redemptive and loving realm. But the man who used to croon "don't escalate" was a memory in my neurons, a few folders of letters, a closet full of old clothes, a never-finished book, and some ashes buried on a hill, lying in a streambed, and remaining in a brown plastic box. He would fear no more the heat of the sun, and fear no more the critics he imagined would tear his book apart. He would yearn no more for reconciliation with Michael, and never again would he make my mother beautiful by telling her so.

VI

GRACE

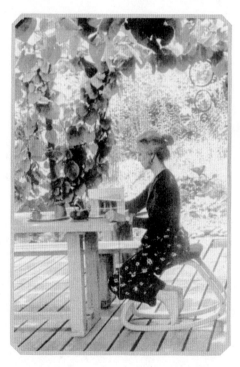

Self-portrait by Valerie Butler, Pine Street, Middletown, Connecticut.

CHAPTER 16

VALERIE MAKES UP HER MIND

My mother and I spent eleven months after my father's death apart, grieving separately. Her life, she said on the phone, felt empty and without meaning. Toni, she said, felt much the same. She repeatedly told me how proud my father had been of me and how much he had loved me. "You and I did a great job taking care of Daddy," she would say. "With your brains and my practical skill, we were a great team!"

I let my hair go gray and cried my way through six free grief counseling sessions offered by my local mental health center. My father's death had marked me, and though I did not wear black, I wanted it to show. I read books about the history of pacemakers, trying to understand what had happened to us, and more books about the health care system. I proposed a story about my father's death to the *New York Times Magazine*. I was haunted by traumatic images of my mother shouting at my father, of his dying, and of our fight at the graveyard on Indian Hill. I did not visit her for Christmas. I was in awe of all she had done for my father, and knew I could not have cared for him nearly as well, and I understood the suffering that led her to be cruel to a man she deeply loved. Yet I was still angry.

In January, to celebrate my sixtieth birthday, I cashed in my frequent-flyer miles, pretended that my father had given me a small legacy (all his assets flowed automatically to my mother), and flew to Bali, where I went repeatedly to a healing water temple called Tirta Empul. Tirta Empul consists of a series of outdoor courtyards surrounded by palm trees. Near the entrance is a long, rectangular stone bath, into which water pours constantly from the mouths of fountains shaped like the heads of gods. I spent a full day there, in a soaked sarong and a traditional white Balinese tunic called a *kebaya,* leaving offerings of flowers and incense by the stone heads and plunging my head under their pouring mouths over and over until my body was chilled, saying to myself, *purify me.* It was as if for seven years I'd slept in a room full of secondhand smoke and at Tirta Empul I finally washed the dirtiness and disgust of my father's death out of my bones.

I came out dazed and changed into dry clothes. The inner courtyards of the temple were crowded with processions of Balinese men and women carrying towers of fruit and flowers on their heads, while others carried the carved god-images they called *barongs* which reminded me of Chinese New Year's dragons. I sat among the crowds, listening to the gentle gonging of the gamelan. It was a holy day, full of life.

At a bar in Ubud, I watched Barack Obama, half a world away, take his first oath of office as president, to cheers all around from Australians and Balinese amazed by the sight of a brown-skinned American president. At an Internet café full of cathode-ray machines, I got an e-mail from an editor at the *New York Times Magazine* saying she was interested in my story about my father, his pacemaker, and the perverse financial incentives within medicine that had encouraged his overtreatment.

My mother stayed put in Middletown. She answered two hundred condolence letters, lifted weights at the Wesleyan gym, and studied tai chi with a new neighbor. She made a few new friends—mainly widowed, divorced, and single women—and decided to go to South Africa to visit a favorite goddaughter, and to get a Siamese cat. She built herself a cat scratcher out of wooden posts and coiled rope, and asked me if I'd take her cat after she died. I lied and promised I would, even though I'm allergic to cats. Then she fainted alone in the house, and did not tell me about it. She simply said she'd decided against going to Africa, and against the cat.

She signed up for a medallion from a company called Lifeline, with a button to summon emergency services. She also went to Dr. Fales's office, signed the forms, and held out her ankle for her own orange plastic DNR bracelet.

"When Jeff's health and mind deteriorated," she wrote in her journal:

> I knew I had to do the hard thing and let him die and not prolong his life with antibiotics, etc. Now as my heart gives me problems I am thinking of the best way to deal with my decline. The thought of going to live in a retirement "home" is simply a horrible idea to me. To be housed, even at The Redwoods, with a lot of old people waiting to die is not my idea of the way to go.

She reread a book she owned called *Last Wish,* in which Betty Rollin describes helping her terminally ill mother take a fatal drug overdose. She told me that she was fantasizing about getting a plastic hose for the exhaust pipe of her car. "There is a prospect of a timely escape," she wrote in her journal, "and I will take it. I need to make things clear to Michael and Jonathan so that Katy does not have the burden of helping me out on her own." I flew east.

On a spring day nearly a year after my father's death, my mother and I drove through a rainstorm to the Longwood Area of Boston, a jumbled maze of traffic-choked streets, streetcar lines, and high-rise hospitals surrounding Harvard Medical School. While walking together in Wesleyan's indoor athletic cage, I'd been shocked to discover that she could not complete a single circuit without stopping to rest. For decades she'd had a heart murmur—a sign that her heart's mitral valve did not close properly—but it had given her no trouble. But the wear and tear of the years had thickened and weakened the valve to the breaking point. In the course of her life, it had opened and closed nearly three billion times. It was flabby and loose, and encrusted with calcium thrown off by her aging bones.

Before going to Boston, she and I visited a Middletown-area cardiologist (not Dr. Rogan) who told her that her aortic valve, too, was stiffened and narrowed. Tapping away on his laptop, he told her to get both heart valves replaced at Yale–New Haven. He wrote down the phone number of a surgeon he trusted and handed it to her, as if that was that.

But rather than calling the number, I did an Internet search and discovered that Brigham and Women's Hospital in Boston, a successor to the old Peter Bent Brigham, was a pioneer in minimally invasive valve replacement surgery. Perhaps, I thought, my mother could have her heart valves replaced without having her breastbone sawed open from the top of her jugular notch at her collarbone to the bottom of her xiphoid process at the base of her ribs.

My mother had good feelings about the Brigham. It was there, in 1971, that she'd gotten her second, possibly life-saving mastectomy under the care of the pioneering surgical chief Francis Daniels Moore. By the time my mother and I returned to the Brigham, however, Moore was only a revered and troubling memory.

He had retired from surgical practice in 1981 at the age of sixty-eight. In his eighties, thanks largely to antibiotics and the safe surgical techniques he'd researched extensively, he survived Legionnaire's disease, two hernia surgeries, and the removal of a benign mass from his pancreas. Then he developed a leaky heart valve and congestive heart failure. The Brigham was a leader in heart surgery in the very elderly, but his doctors did not think he was a good candidate for it, and put him on medication. Short of breath, he lived a constricted and declining life.

In the late fall of 2001—a month, as it happened, after my father's first stroke—Moore shot himself to death in the study of his home in the Boston suburb of Westwood. He was eighty-eight. His death was traumatic, bloody, and old-fashioned. And in wresting control of its timing and manner from the advanced medicine that he helped create, Moore remained the hero of his own journey. My mother, I suspected, would want the same.

I was nervous and preoccupied as we arrived at the hospital, and not just by the rain pouring in sheets off the windshield. On our drive from Middletown, just after pulling out of a tollbooth onto the Massachusetts Turnpike, my mother abruptly stopped the car in the active right lane of traffic, seemingly oblivious to the danger, to turn over the wheel to me. As I hurried into the driver's seat, looking over my shoulder at a truck slowly accelerating out of the tollbooth behind us, I wondered for the first time whether her mind was starting to slip.

I'd earlier sent her an article I found in the *New York Times*, headlined, "Saving the Heart Can Sometimes Mean Losing the

Memory." It suggested that somewhere between a tenth and a half of heart bypass patients tested poorly on memory and other thinking skills six months after surgery. Other studies suggested that the deficits persisted for years. Doctors sometimes called the phenomenon "pump head" because it was popularly thought to affect people who'd been hooked up to a heart-lung bypass pump, even though patients who had joint replacements and other major surgeries also suffered similar mental declines. Some doctors speculated that in heart patients the brain damage occurred when surgeons clamped and unclamped the aorta, the body's largest blood vessel, breaking up the coating of fat and calcium inside it and dislodging a snowstorm of tiny clots that traveled through the bloodstream to the brain. The clamping could also dislodge larger clots: many studies show that 2 to 5 percent of those undergoing heart surgery suffer strokes as well.

I had other fears that I did not share. Earlier that year, the eighty-seven-year-old mother of a close California friend named Christie had taken three gruesome months to die in Florida after being shuttled back and forth repeatedly between a hospital and a nursing home. She'd been rushed into valve replacement surgery by her doctor, and Christie, to her later regret, had pressed her mother to overcome her reluctance and go ahead. The surgical shock had been too much.

We entered Brigham and Women's through a dark and bustling front entrance. The place had the disjointed, eternally-under-construction feel of a modern airport. We rode up an escalator and crossed an airy pedestrian bridge into the soaring Carl J. and Ruth Shapiro Cardiovascular Center, an uplifting place, almost like a cathedral, with windows three stories high. The only decrepit things in the place were some of the patients: they sat in their upholstered chairs in various states of health and illness, some in wheelchairs or trundling canisters of oxygen.

*   *   *

We sat in a windowless treatment room and waited. When the surgeon came in and asked us why we were there, my mother said, "To ask questions." She was no longer a trusting and deferential patient. Like me, she no longer saw doctors—perhaps with the exception of her internist, Dr. Fales—as healers or her fiduciaries. They were skilled technicians with their own agendas. But I couldn't help feeling that something precious—our old faith in a doctor's calling, perhaps, or in a healing that is more than a financial transaction or a reflexive fixing of broken parts—had been lost.

The surgeon told us that my mother's age—she was eighty-four—was not a barrier. In the 1950s, when heart-valve surgery was risky and experimental, doctors, by tacit agreement, did not think of operating on people much over fifty. But in the 1970s, after the advent of efficient heart-lung machines, reliable Medicare reimbursements, and safer surgical techniques, the average age of heart-valve patients began to rise. By 2008, when my mother and I arrived there, a quarter of Brigham and Women's heart-valve patients were over eighty.

The surgeon was forthright: without open-heart surgery, there was a fifty-fifty chance my mother would die within two years. If she survived the operation, she would probably live to be ninety—the normal life expectancy for a woman of her age. And the risks? He shrugged. Six to eight weeks at least of recovery. A 5 percent chance of stroke. Some possibility, he acknowledged at my prompting, of postoperative cognitive decline.

My mother lifted her trouser leg to reveal her anklet of orange plastic: the DNR bracelet. The doctor recoiled. No, he would not operate with that bracelet in place. It would not be fair to his team. She would be revived if she collapsed. She would spend time recovering in intensive care. "If I have a stroke," my mother said, nearly in tears, "I want you to let me go." What about a minor stroke, the doctor said—a little weakness on one side?

I kept my mouth shut. I was there to get her the information she needed and to support whatever decision she made. If she emerged from surgery intellectually damaged, I would bring her to The Redwoods in California and try to care for her the way she had cared for my father at such a cost to her own health. The thought terrified me.

The doctor sent her up a floor for an echocardiogram. I went into the waiting room, called my brother Jonathan, and let loose my fears. Half an hour later, my mother came back and put on her black coat. "No," she said brightly, with the clarity of purpose she had shown when she asked me to have my father's pacemaker deactivated. "I will not do it."

CHAPTER 17

OLD PLUM TREE
BENT AND GNARLED

M y mother spent her last spring and summer arranging house repairs, thinning out my father's bookcases with Toni's help, and throwing out the files he collected for the book he never finished writing, saving only the love letters he'd written her when they were in their sixties. She told Toni that she didn't want to leave a mess for her kids.

"I must get right with Michael," she wrote in her journal. "I am so saddened by his refusal to visit—so distant and doesn't call, or when I do call is in a hurry to go somewhere. Not good." Finally he called and proposed coming to see her, but when he said he wanted her to pay for a rental car, she balked and he exploded. "I must work on forgiveness," she wrote in her journal, after writing down the wounding things he'd said. "It will only corrode me. I feel abandoned and alone." She sent me a DVD about forgiveness, hoping I'd pass it on to him, but I didn't dare.

In her journal she wrote about my father with a tenderness she could not express while she was caring for him. "I'm overwhelmed by sadness missing the old Jeff as I knew him—his wit and compassion and his sheer liveliness. Oh God how I miss him now."

"All quiet," she wrote on a Monday in May. "I spent the morning in Jeff's study sorting out boxes and boxes of research so lovingly collected by my poor darling." Her chest pain worsened, and her breathlessness grew severe. "I'm aching to garden, to tidy up the neglect of my major achievement," she wrote. "Without it the place would be so ordinary and dull. But so it goes. ACCEPT ACCEPT ACCEPT."

In July, she went to a new cardiologist, a partner in Dr. Rogan's group practice, for a second opinion. He said she might have severe coronary artery disease as well as stiff and leaky heart valves, and suggested she consider a less invasive operation: the insertion of stents to prop open the partially blocked arteries in her heart, an operation that might reduce her chest pain. He also suggested she consider an experimental valve replacement, performed by floating the device down a vein. "When I mentioned stroke risk," he wrote in his clinical notes, "she immediately was turned off and did not want to pursue further discussion, again desiring only palliative care." He thought she'd been unnecessarily frightened by the doctor at Brigham and Women's.

I sent her a copy of *Dr. Dean Ornish's Program for Reversing Heart Disease,* which advocated a vegan, nonfat diet. I found out online that Middlesex Hospital offered a meditation class in mindfulness-based stress reduction, based on the teachings of Jon Kabat-Zinn, whose CD my mother listened to every morning. I also discovered that Middlesex offered a "heart nurse" program to help her manage her physical symptoms—something none of her doctors had referred her to—and I got her to sign up for both. Peaches, Jonathan's long-ago girlfriend whom my mother had embraced as a surrogate daughter and who was now a Unitarian-Universalist minister, came to visit from Vermont.

I did not go.

She deserved better from me, and now it is too late.

My mother's heart nurse called me, urging me to get my mother to reconsider surgery. My mother was so healthy in other ways, the nurse said. I called Dr. Dennis McCullough, a geriatrics doctor and leading pioneer of Slow Medicine in the United States. "Eighty-four is still relatively young," he said. Uneasy, I called Dr. Fales.

"I know your mother well enough, and I respect her," he said. "She doesn't want to risk a surgery that could leave her debilitated or bound for a nursing home. I think I would make the same decision if it was my mom." I called my mother and said, "Are you sure? The surgeon said you could live to be ninety."

"I don't want to live to be ninety," she said.

"I'm going to miss you," I said, weeping. "You are not only my mother. You are my friend."

That August, she had a heart attack. I was away that weekend and heard the news via Michael, whom she'd called from the hospital when she could not reach me. He gave her low-key, empathic support over the phone. He told me she wanted to funnel all communication through him: she apparently needed his quiet empathy more than my activist fixing. She was still in the hospital, in a step-down unit after several days in intensive care, when I got a call from yet another member of Middlesex Cardiology Associates, who'd been handed my mother's case. The desire of doctors not to give up on my mother, to resist death, and to show their caring by doing something, anything, seemed unstoppable.

The doctor had gotten the results back from a cardiac catheterization, an invasive and stressful test with risks of its own, for which they'd threaded a long tube from her groin into her heart, injected dye into her arteries, and taken X-rays. The news was bad. The worst of the narrowing in her heart vessels was in places too difficult to stent.

Instead, the doctors were considering giving my mother coronary artery bypass grafts plus the two valve-replacement surgeries she'd rejected when she had a far better chance of surviving open-heart surgery in decent shape. My mother seemed to be heading down the greased chute toward a series of "Hail Mary" surgeries—risky, painful, dangerous, and harrowing, each one increasing the chance that her death, when it came, would take place in intensive care. The cost to Medicare would probably have been in the $80,000 to $150,000 range, with higher payments if things had not gone well. More than a third of Medicare patients have surgery in their last year of life, nearly a tenth have surgery in the last month of life, and a fifth die in intensive care. Medical overtreatment costs the U.S. health care system an estimated $158 billion to $226 billion a year.

Burning with anger, I told the astonished cardiologist that my mother had rejected surgery before her heart attack and I saw no reason to subject her to it now. My intuitive revulsion, I would later discover, had a basis in medical evidence: one major study found that 13 percent of patients over eighty who underwent combined valve and bypass surgeries died in the hospital. In a smaller, confirming study, 13 percent died in the hospital and an additional 40 percent were discharged to nursing homes.

I called my mother in her hospital bed.

"I think we're grasping . . ." I stopped.

"At straws," she finished my sentence. She was quiet.

"It's hard," she said, "to give up hope."

Four hours later she called me back. "I want you to give my sewing machine to a woman who really sews. It's a Bernina. They don't make them like this any more. It's all metal, no plastic parts."

"But I'd like it," I said.

"But Katy," she said. "You don't sew."

I said, "You're right."

I called her the next day. "I'm ready to die," she said, seemingly unaware of Michael's continuing ambivalence. "I'm at peace with all my children." She was overflowing. She told me she'd found the little spiral-bound book I made her for her eightieth birthday. "It was so loving," she said, "And oh, Katy, I didn't appreciate it."

"Cherish Brian," she went on.

"You mean, stop being a snob and cherish Brian?" I asked.

"That's exactly what I mean. I *love* Brian," she said. "I *love* Brian for what he's done for you."

An old Zen master once wrote:

Old plum tree bent and gnarled
all at once opens one blossom, two blossoms,
three, four, five blossoms, uncountable blossoms . . .
Whirling, changing into wind, wild rain,
falling, snow, all over the earth.

My mother was like that.

My brother Jonathan brought her home from the hospital with a portable oxygen tank. Tests had shown that her heart was damaged badly enough to qualify her for hospice care. She could no longer walk upstairs on her own without fainting, and Jonathan oversaw the installation of a stair glide—that informal harbinger of impending death—like the ones my father and Brian's father had used for a few months. Peaches visited. I explored getting counseling at my local hospice, but decided not to when I learned that because my mother was dying on the other side of the country and not as one of their clients, I didn't qualify for Medicare-covered services and would have to pay out of pocket.

A week later, Jonathan flew back to his truck-driving job, and Michael, further renouncing decades of self-protection, flew in while I kept writing. My mother cooked for him and washed his dishes. They had a classic, familiar fight, set off by her attempt to limit how much roast chicken he ate—a fight so intense that he called me and asked me to book him an immediate flight back to California. I said I would, but suggested he wait a few hours. With help from a hospice social worker conducting shuttle diplomacy, he and my mother began talking again, this time in earnest, and with care. He spoke to her for hours about the pain of their intense, difficult relationship, stretching back to his childhood. "I had no idea," she said, when he was done. "I can't fix it. All I can do is listen and acknowledge."

She updated her will. She copied out a line from Helen Keller on a three-by-five card: "The best and most beautiful things in the world cannot be seen or even touched—they must be felt with the heart." A hospice nurse cut off her long beautiful white hair, because she was now too weak to shower or wash it on her own. She took digitalis and squirted morphine under her tongue when she needed to manage her intense heart pain. She needed more care than her struggling son or the limited nursing hours provided by the underfunded hospice program could give her.

She needed someone there all the time. She needed me. But she did not say, "I need you," and like a fool, or a workaholic, or a human being in denial, I did not have the sense to simply go. Nobody lectured me on my moral obligations, as my Victorian great-grandfather James might have done.

My mother watched a moth emerge from a chrysalis brought over by a neighbor child and took her last photograph of its wet crumpled wings. She took out her calligraphy pens and wrote out a poem by the ancient Chinese sage Wu-Men for Brian's upcoming birthday:

Ten thousand flowers in spring, the moon in autumn,
a cool breeze in summer, snow in winter.
If your mind isn't clouded by unnecessary things,
this is the best season of your life.

Then, on a small piece of paper, she brushed out her final circular *enso* and wrote beneath it, "For my memorial service."

Sitting under the fig tree in my California garden, I felt something descend from the sky and pour through me like grace. "Your mother is dying," said a voice inside my heart. "This is a sacred time." With the support of my editor, I decided to abandon my nearly finished article and fly to Connecticut. The phone rang. It was Michael, calling from Pine Street. He and our mother, he said, were continuing to talk. There was more to resolve, he wanted more time alone with her, and she, he said, wanted it too. I called an old colleague of my father's in Middletown. My mother was still full of beans, he said, and had even gotten up from the couch, trailing her oxygen tube, to make him a martini. She would probably last months. I deferred to my brother, ignored my heart, and pushed back my flight.

Three days later, I called her. I'd just come home from my local bookstore, where a former student had read from his new book about the ritual of tea, and I couldn't stop thinking of her. I remembered how she'd swirl boiling water into her beloved Japanese iron teapot to warm it, pour it out and add fresh hot water and loose tea, putting on the lid and tucking the pot under the indigo-blue tea cozy she'd sewn herself. I remembered her attentively setting out thin white bone china cups for my father and me, and a white plate holding six fanned ginger snaps. I remembered how, no matter how badly things were going, we'd gather each day at the kitchen table—waiting as the tea steeped, enjoying one another, and simply being alive. Then the ritual drinking of the tea itself, making us relaxed and alert at the same time.

But I had been too defensive and clumsy, too afraid of her criticism, and too much of a feminist bookworm to learn from her how to do this.

In an outpouring, I told her all this. She was the one who could get through a meal without reading the paper; she was the one who got up at dawn to meditate when things with my father got rough; she was the one who put her compassion into action and honored her vows and took care of the man she'd loved.

"But Katy," she said, her voice weak, after I finally stopped talking. "You are yourself. You're good at other things."

Then she said, "There isn't much time."

That night she could not stop vomiting. She was taken to the hospital with Michael following the ambulance in her white Camry. "Don't call your siblings," she told him when they got to the hospice unit. "They'll only panic and come."

Eihei Dogen, the great Buddhist teacher who revitalized Zen in Japan in the twelfth century, had these words to say about dying: "In birth there is nothing but birth and in death there is nothing but death. Accordingly, when birth comes, become and manifest birth, and when death comes, become and manifest death. Do not avoid them or desire them."

My mother died like that.

She told the hospice nurses that she wanted to stop eating and drinking, that she wanted to die and never go home. Her heart-management nurse stopped by her bed and said she hoped this was just a bump in the road. My mother said, "It feels like an avalanche." She had dry heaves and could not catch her breath. She took off her hammered silver earrings, and said, "I want to get rid of all the garbage." She told Michael to call Jonathan and me. By the time he came back from the phone, she was dead. He broke into sobs.

It could have been too much self-administered morphine or too little potassium. It could have been the stress of the cardiac catheterization. It could have been getting up and making martinis for the people who stopped by to see her. In the end, does it matter?

She died of old age, sickness, and death. She died of a heart calcified and broken by six years of nonstop caregiving. She died of being eighty-four. She was continent and lucid to her end. She took back her body from her doctors. She died the death she chose, not the death they had in mind. She reclaimed her moral authority from the broken medical system that had held her husband hostage. She died like a warrior. Her dying was painful, messy, and imperfect, but that is the uncontrollable nature of dying. She faced it head-on. My brother Jonathan called it a triumph.

I would have liked to sit with her body in her hospice room, or brought her home to her house on Pine Street one last time and put her in the living room in a plain wooden coffin surrounded by candles, the way the family managed it for my great-grandfather James. I wanted to wash her body in sweet tea, the way her friend the Zen priest Issan Dorsey did with the bodies of young men who died of AIDS in the 1980s. I would have liked to care for my mother's body as freely as did the poorest peasant in a straw-thatched hut in Ireland in the nineteenth century.

But we had no rituals to follow by rote in our numbness; hospitals run on schedules, patients need beds, and Medicare does not reimburse for care to the dead. Funeral homes have rules, as do states. In Connecticut, a body cannot be released to anyone but a funeral director. By the time my flight landed, my mother's body had been gurneyed to a freezer in the hospital basement. Over the weekend, the morgue staff would call us repeatedly to urge us to move it out, just as Discharge Planning had pressured us, eight years earlier, to quickly move my stroke-ridden father to a rehabilitation center.

My brothers and I settled on the funeral home on Long Island Sound where my father's body had become white ashes a year and a half earlier. We had to threaten to take our business elsewhere to get them to allow us to be with her body for ten minutes, and to put flowers in her cardboard bier, before it was consigned to the flames.

Cremation remains an industrial rather than a hallowed process. We would have to sneak any sense of the sacred into the cracks. The cremation worker, whose name we did not know, was quiet and treated us with sensitivity. There was no ceremonial lighting of the gas pilot, as there is a ceremonial tossing of the first spade of dirt onto the coffin. There was no chanting of "ashes to ashes, and dust to dust." There was nothing like the beauty I'd seen in Bali, where I saw the bones of the dead placed in the stomach of a heavy, black-painted wooden bull and paraded through the streets on the backs of relatives and villagers, to a park where the gamelan played for the crowds and the flames were lit.

We put lilies in the cardboard box that held her, but we could not prettify her death. We'd asked the funeral home to dress her in her scarlet silk *ao dai,* but someone had put it on backward. The fabric stretched awkwardly across her maimed chest, and the delicately knotted frogs she'd fashioned herself lay unbuttoned at the back of her neck. Now that she was stiff we could not make it right. Her mouth was pulled to one side. Her hair was shorn. Her skin was gray. The beauty and elegance that had awed and intimidated me all my life was gone. She was naked of the silver earrings and bracelets she'd always worn, then dangling from my own ears and wrist. For the first time that I could remember, I was not afraid of her.

I did not feel at peace with her death the way I'd felt at peace with my father's. She died too soon for my taste—though not for hers—just as my father had died too late. My good-byes felt incomplete. I wanted to ask for her forgiveness, or better yet, to turn back the clock and care for her more tenderly during her final year. But time moves forward, not back. We had done our best. We had expressed, in our own peculiar and broken ways, our love. She had not been a perfect mother. I had not been a perfect daughter. It had not been a perfect death. I would never live a perfect life.

Jonathan, Michael, and I watched through a plate-glass window as the cardboard box containing the remnants of our mother's fine body, stripped of its temporal beauty, slid into the flames. The next day, the undertaker would deliver a brown plastic box to the house on Pine Street where, for forty-five of their sixty-one years together, my parents had loved and looked after each other, humanly and imperfectly. There were no bits of metal mixed with the fine white powder and small pieces of her bones.

After her memorial service, I would fly home and learn to say to Brian, "I need you" and "I love you." I would undress my sixty-year-old body in front of him, and hear him praise my beauty, just as my father had done for my mother when she was my age. I would wear my mother's worn Japanese cotton bathrobe, bought decades earlier on one of our trips to Tassajara, until it fell in strips from my shoulders. I would wear shoes that she'd bought at Marshalls during my father's death watch, a half-size too small for me, until they gave me a painful corn.

I would vow that in the future I would not wait for the imminence of death to say, *I love you, thank you, please forgive me, I forgive you, good-bye.* I would settle her estate, take down her photographs and the whorl of dried sticks she'd hung over the fireplace, and give my brother Jonathan her Bernina sewing machine and my brother Michael a quilt she'd sewn of patches of Japanese indigo, under which she and my father once slept. I would find her long silk underwear in a drawer, and finally understand how she'd stayed warm while keeping the heat turned down so low that I was always freezing. I'd sell her beautiful house on Pine Street to a couple who would set up the husband's Lionel train set in the basement where my father had labored over his unfinished book.

I would distribute the inheritance she preserved for her children by keeping her husband out of a nursing home. Still driven by our rivalry for the love of the dead, my brothers and I would fight over things that seem trivial now, and I would discover that I would need to ask for people's forgiveness, for things big and small, until the day I died, because I am human. I would soften my heart. I would commit to Brian in a way I couldn't when I stood in the long corridor of my parents' dying.

On the first anniversary of my mother's death, I would borrow a Jewish ritual, buy a twenty-four-hour *Yahrzeit* candle from the kosher section at Safeway, and put it, with a vase of flowers, next to a wooden Buddha from Thailand that my mother had given me long ago. I would set up photographs of my parents, one of her looking glamorous at Ben Carton's wedding, and another of her raking leaves in her beloved garden while my grinning father happily wields a rented leaf blower. I would bring beauty and ceremony to their memories in ways I had not known how to do when they lay dying. I would pin to my bulletin board a photograph of my mother and me holding each other in bed, remember her softly calling me "Sweetie," and loosen my grip on the story I'd long told, that she never loved me. I would cry, no longer afraid to love her and to miss her, no longer afraid to walk toward her, knowing that my tears and sadness were the beautiful flip side of the bright coin of love and of acceptance of the imperfect. I would stay close to my eighty-year-old neighbor after he had a minor stroke, and stand prepared to help him and his wife further when the time came. I would no longer put all my life's coins into the basket of work and allow my fears to hold me back from loving. I would cherish Brian. I would work the glass splinter out of my heart. I would remain myself.

In time the things I brought home from Pine Street and

fetishized with my longings—her more-than-a-lifetime supply of Swiss cotton nightgowns, a hand-embroidered purple sash, even her leftover hair gel and CVS cold cream—would become nothing more than things. I would emerge from my time in the half-light and leave behind the liminal world between life and death, where I had dwelt so long with my parents. I would stop trying, like Orpheus with his lyre, to lead my mother's shade out of the underworld, to sing her up from the depths into the light. I would die as a dutiful daughter and be reborn as some sort of grown-up whom I could not yet define. On Saturday mornings I would steam half-and-half and make Brian coffee and bring it up to him, along with a cup of green tea for me and the *New York Times,* and we would lie for hours together, intimate and luxurious. I would walk on my mountain in the spring, and laugh with my friends, and become happier and more grateful for my remaining life than I had ever been.

I would find among my parents' things a photograph taken by Toni not long after she first came to work for us. In it, my arms are flung protectively around my parents' shoulders, my hair is shiny and brown, and I am grinning broadly, while my mother looks away from the camera exhausted, and my father wears his chronic post-stroke mask of surprised confusion. Gray-haired now, and nearly ten years older, I would whisper, "Poor Jeff," shaking my head in sorrow over his final years of unnecessary suffering. I would regret many things I'd done and left undone, as do most of the dutiful daughters and sons I know, but I would never feel guilty for having tried to turn off his pacemaker or for beating back my mother's doctors, with greater success, when they seemed bent on stretching out the stub end of her life. I would understand that things that look heartless to outsiders must sometimes be done out of love.

All of that was to come.

VII

INTO
THE LIGHT

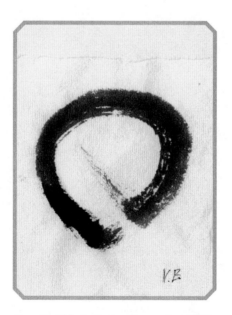

Enso by Valerie Butler, September 2009.
Left with a note: "For my memorial service."

CHAPTER 18

A BETTER WAY OF DEATH

By working creatively, and in ways yet
unthought of, the lobby of the dying and the
gravely ill could become a healing force in
society.

—IVAN ILLICH, *Medical Nemesis*

On Father's Day 2010, two years after my father's death and
nearly a year after my mother's, Brian and I had friends
over for brunch beneath our backyard fig tree. It was a sunny
green Sunday in late June. That day the *New York Times Magazine* published the story I'd written about my father and his
pacemaker, and I was afraid that my mother and I would come
across to readers as heartless.

During brunch, my e-mail in-box filled up with messages.
When I turned on my computer around noon, "What Broke My
Father's Heart: How a Pacemaker Wrecked Our Family's Life"
was at the top of the *Times*'s most-e-mailed list. By the time
the weekend was over, more than seventeen hundred people
had responded, either by e-mailing me directly or by posting
comments on the *Times*'s Web site. The messages—from doc-

tors, nurses, elderly people, and baby boomers with aging parents—came from across the United States and from Australia, India, Ireland, Italy, Saudi Arabia, and the Netherlands. The sheer volume made clear how deep uneasiness runs over medicine's current default response to death. A cardiologist in Italy summed up the tone of many: "What happened to your parents was horrible, and your mother did the right thing." I felt as if I were listening in on the first reveal of a vast, previously unvoiced public conversation.

"I have never been a big reader & certainly not the *New York Times*," e-mailed a registered nurse from Minnesota. "I am feeling a little self-conscious about writing to you." Her passion was working with people over eighty, she said, and she had watched "the suffering, lack of dignity & overall poor quality of life they experience. Every day at some point someone says to me, 'I just want to die. I have lived my life, it's enough.'"

One family, she said, had recently notified her agency that they agreed to a pacemaker for their elderly father with late-stage dementia after doctors told them it would improve his memory and quality of life. "I felt like dying inside," the nurse went on:

> I could not tell them what I really think, since the procedure was done & they were misled. . . . It is so frustrating for me how some physicians are not ok with death & dying & are usually too afraid to even discuss this natural process. Instead they want to save everyone's lives & not provide choice.

A woman from Malaysia said my parents would not have suffered so badly had my brothers and I helped more. Some doctors felt I'd unfairly painted them as money-driven and said that fear of litigation, in the face of insistence and denial by families, drove much overtreatment. Other doctors, however, were troubled by the drift of their profession. "I am often disturbed by the unnecessary interventions I see being performed all around me," said a Texas surgeon on the *Times*'s Web site. "These doctors are not bad people, they are simply used to 'knee-jerk' fixes for piecemeal problems, rather than a clear discussion of what the ultimate goals of treatment really are." A Philadelphia doctor added:

> Both my parents, and dozens of patients who I attended to, have suffered through this maze as well. I am a physician and a son who struggled, without much guidance twenty years ago to know when to gain acceptance of what is really an inevitable, natural part of our human existence. Thank you for the tears, water clarifies.

A woman described the unforeseen consequences of a hip-replacement surgery given a seventy-nine-year-old relative who was in the early stages of dementia. "When she never recovered from the addle-minded state immediately following anesthesia, we were told, 'Oh yes, some patients never really get their cognitive abilities back.' THANKS FOR TELLING US. So much for an informed decision!"

Another had tried to decline a pacemaker for a demented mother living in a nursing home. "The surgeon called me and said he was putting the case to the hospital ethics committee and I would have to deal with them," she wrote me:

> He was quite rude, indignant, guilt provoking and you know the rest. I reluctantly folded and let the doctor proceed. Yesterday was my mother's eighty-ninth birthday. She does not know me. She does not dress herself. She wears diapers. Her hair is falling out, her face is mottled with horrible looking spots, her ankles are swollen and she weighs 109 pounds at 5 feet 7 inches. Why did I ever allow that pacemaker to be implanted?

*   *   *

A month later, my phone rang. It was a woman whom I didn't know, a yoga therapist named Bella McCloud, calling from central California. For two years, she'd been the full-time caregiver for her demented father, first in the home she shared with her husband and their blended family of four children, and then, when the stress on everyone grew too much, in a unit in a duplex she owned nearby. Her father began waking multiple times at night, and so did she as he paced the floors looking for the bathroom and sometimes, in his confusion, peed on the kitchen floor. Exhausted, she knew that her health and stamina would soon give out and that the only alternative would be to put him in a skilled nursing facility, where he would probably be sedated to control his wandering, or even restrained. A year earlier, she'd asked her father's cardiologist about turning off her dad's pacemaker, but had gotten a mystifying, paradoxical answer that added up to a *no*: on the one hand, the device *could not be* deactivated because her father might die immediately without it; on the other hand, it *didn't need to be* deactivated, because it wouldn't keep him alive when he was ready to die.

Then she read my article online. She called her father's primary care doctor, and the two women met at the local emergency room to arrange to have him admitted to the hospital. After his doctor said, "We are going to turn off the pacemaker," hospital staff questioned her orders for the first time in her career. The case was referred to the hospital bioethics committee. After extensive interviews with Bella, the doctor, and others, the committee ruled that deactivating the pacemaker would be "kind and compassionate."

Bella, who is working on a memoir about her experience, had a conversation with her father, who had been talking more and more frequently about people he loved who were long dead. It went something like this:

Do you miss your (late) mom and dad?
Yes.
Do you miss your (late) wife?
Yes.
Would you like to be with them?
Yes.
Do you know how to get there?
No.
Would you like me to help you?
Yes.

Bella, who was her father's legally appointed medical decision-maker, took him back to her duplex. A team from the device manufacturer came out and, after some hesitation, deactivated the device. Bella and her daughter pushed two beds together in the living room, in front of a window overlooking the ocean, and stayed with her father as he grew weaker, sleeping with him throughout the night, their hands entwined with his, heads resting together. He died peacefully, one week and one hour after the pacemaker was disabled, in her home, in her arms, surrounded with love. Thanks to his daughter's extraordinary efforts, medical overdoing was undone, and he died the Good Death that our ancestors so prized—in the bosom of family, at home, and in a state of acceptance. It was an expression of a new Art of Dying for a biotechnical time: one requiring discernment, resisting Fast Medicine's default never-quit pathway, and honoring death.

The decision was Slow Medicine at its best—a shared decision that took into account the suffering of the whole family and did not focus reflexively on fixing an organ or extending a life.

It empowered the people who carried the burden rather than doctors who would perform a heroic intervention and then leave the family to pick up the pieces. It accepted the reality of her father's twin terminal illnesses—dementia and heart trouble. It was not made in isolation by an exhausted daughter but with the support and validation of a larger moral community. It was the fruit of unusually harmonious cooperation between a family and a medical institution. It was, in its own way, loving, beautiful, and holy.

This is one possible path to death.

Not long afterward, Brian and I watched another death, one that showed me that the problem of American dying has causes far deeper than perverse economic incentives within medicine. The problem lies also with our culture, which is unwilling to engage with death until it is in our faces. One of Brian's closest friends, a hardy, healthy fifty-nine-year-old Colorado River guide and specialist in the alternative-medicine approach called homeopathy, was suddenly overcome by seizures and vomiting. At the hospital, doctors diagnosed a fatal melanoma that had metastasized to many internal organs, including his liver, bowels, and spleen. There were signs of eleven tumors in his brain alone. We watched in horror as David turned down any suggestion of hospice and insisted instead that everything be done, no matter how bad the odds. He had weeks of whole-brain radiation and then a last-ditch "Hail Mary" neurosurgery. The neurosurgeon, who met David face-to-face for the first time after he was already prepped for surgery, could not guarantee that the operation had even a fifty-fifty chance of helping him and acknowledged there were risks it would make him worse. David insisted. He entered surgery able to talk, walk, e-mail, and make his own decisions. He woke up unable to formulate a sentence, in diapers, and unable to walk or to complete the emotional work necessary for a Good Death. In that condition he died, nine weeks after his cancer diagnosis.

Consider, too, a common pathway to a living death, this one traversed by eighty-four-year-old Marguerite Wolff, the mother of journalist Michael Wolff. She'd been having fainting spells, and by the time she was taken from her assisted living complex to the hospital for heart-valve surgery, she was already too forgetful to live on her own, count, organize a Thanksgiving dinner, or tell time. She came out of her surgery with a perfectly fixed-up heart, almost psychotic levels of agitation, a tendency to roam and to hit, and cascading losses of memory and language. She was soon evicted from assisted living for needing too much assistance and placed under twenty-four-hour care, paid for by her children, in a rented Manhattan apartment. She had seizures and became mute, unable to walk, and relentlessly angry, with one ancient path to a merciful death—a slowly failing heart—thoroughly blocked. "My siblings and I must take the blame here," Wolff wrote in 2012 in *New York* magazine, belatedly reflecting on their barely pondered decision to approve surgery rather than face the prospect of their mother's mortality. "It did not once occur to us to say: 'You want to do major heart surgery on an eighty-four-year-old woman showing progressive signs of dementia? What are you, nuts?'"

Consider, finally, the death of Kenneth Harris Krieger, a retired engineer, who died the way many of us die now. In the summer of 2011, when he was eighty-eight and too demented to remember how to rake leaves, he came down with a bloodstream infection of mysterious origin. His daughter Lisa, a science reporter for the *San Jose Mercury News,* rushed him from his assisted living residence to the emergency room. He had signed a do-not-resuscitate order and wanted to die a natural death, but nobody had prepared his daughter for the practical implications of carrying out those wishes. She had never considered palliative care or hospice, and she was alone. Nobody viewed her as a patient in addition to her father. She hadn't accepted the coming of death.

Her father was treated at Stanford Hospital, nationally famous for its pioneering work in heart transplantation. In consultation with Lisa, doctors there decided that his do-not-resuscitate order did not prohibit them from sending her father to the intensive care unit and attaching him to a respirator to buy him enough time for antibiotics to work. He was sedated, and Lisa never again saw her father conscious.

The drugs didn't work. Each decision after that, as his daughter wrote for her newspaper in February 2012, was "incremental": another drug, another problem, another treatment, another test, another organ system in failure, another stratospherically expensive drug. By the time her father died ten days later, after Lisa refused to permit a last-ditch surgery to remove gangrenous tissue destroyed by a rampant infection of strep bacteria called necrotizing fasciitis, he had been subjected to $323,000 worth of painful medical treatment, including $25,000 a day for his ICU bed and $48,000 for a single day's dosing with immunoglobulin. (Most of the expense was absorbed or cost-shifted by Stanford.) He was moved to a hospice bed and died without ever regaining consciousness.

Lisa never got to say good-bye to her father the way I'd been blessed to say good-bye to mine. She went on to write powerful articles about the botched end of his life and about advanced medical directives and palliative care. Her father's was not an unusual path to death—the panicked trip to the emergency room, the family members unprepared, hundreds of thousands in public and private dollars wasted, the implications of his DNR and his dementia ignored, and doctors who'd never previously met the family busily deploying painful forms of futility rather than facing the reality of an old man's dying and speaking the truth. It was a death by Fast Medicine—protracted, expensive, and traumatic. And it is almost nobody's idea of a Good Death.

Reclaiming death from medicine, the way the natural childbirth movement recaptured birth in the 1970s, is already underway in the form of open rebellion by families like mine; the growth of hospice and palliative-care programs; and the widening numbers of doctors who practice Slow Medicine—though they may not call it that—especially in geriatrics and primary care and in critical care, pulmonology, cardiology, and oncology.

But the economic forces arrayed against reclaiming the deathbed are immense. Reimbursements for advanced medical technologies, which become forms of medical torture when inappropriately deployed, help cover the cost of a sales representative's mortgage payments, a hospital's money-losing emergency room, a surgeon's second or third home, or dividends to stockholders of Siemens or St. Jude Medical. Nothing much will change until we pay doctors and hospitals when they appropriately do less as well as we do when they inappropriately do too much.

One physician told me that if he relied only on Medicare reimbursements for his rotations on the palliative-care service—which were essentially subsidized by his salary from a university hospital research post—he would earn about $40,000 a year working full-time. An oncologist who spends an hour or more having a truthful conversation with a distraught family about the dim prospects of yet another round of chemotherapy for a metastasized cancer will barely be compensated. One who goes ahead with an untested, harrowing, and dubious drug, sometimes against his best judgment, will have to spend less time per patient and will be better financially rewarded, even getting a markup on the cost of the drug itself. If a cardiac surgeon ventures a "Hail Mary" surgery on a very sick patient with multiple fatal illnesses, perhaps in her last month of life, he and the hospital will be paid more by Medicare than if he performs the same operation on a healthier patient with a more reasonable chance for long-term survival.

Doctors are often insulted by the suggestion that such financial strictures help shape their medical treatment, but just as surely as the home-mortgage deduction promotes home ownership, economic incentives and disincentives—along with discomfort with dying, fear of being sued or accused of conducting "death panels," and feelings of professional failure—encourage specialists to refer patients to hospice care only days before death, essentially dumping them on the program for morphine drips after wringing out every last expensive procedure from their suffering bodies. This helps explain why half of people who die under hospice care spend eighteen days or less there, when they could have benefited from up to six months of its physical, spiritual, emotional, and practical help.

Changes in Medicare's reimbursement structure could help. Perhaps someday Medicare will offer us the choice of a "Plan Q" covering up to two years of home and palliative care in exchange for the willingness not to expect Medicare to pay for a last-ditch $35,000 defibrillator, a futile and debilitating surgery for an incurable brain tumor, a $50,000 chemotherapy buying only a couple of pain-wracked months, a $300,000 ICU death, or a $500,000 external heart pump. Perhaps we will look with more humility on the British National Health Service, which gives better home support to its chronically ill elderly, but doesn't cover drugs and procedures that string out dying if they cost more than $50,000 per year of life gained. Perhaps someday we will have the spine to admit that people routinely die in hospitals and will push for protocols for humane care there, like Britain's Liverpool Care Pathway for the Dying Patient. Perhaps someday we will have an "811" number to bring a flying squad of palliative care and hospice doctors and nurses to the home to provide reassurance to the panicked family and pain management to the dying, as an alternative to a brutal final tour through 911, the ER, and the ICU.

Changes like these are unlikely to come without a grass-roots movement of doctors and family caregivers advocating Slow Medicine—humane, realistic, appropriate, not always cheaper, and sometimes time-consuming (but not technology-consuming) medical care for the last phase of life. The antidote for overtreatment is not undertreatment: it's appropriate care. When the body can no longer be healed, there can still be healing for the family—and for the soul.

As the caregiving crisis deepens, perhaps a grassroots family-caregivers' movement will fight for better funding for such care. Perhaps it will counterbalance the powerful health care industry lobby, made up of hospitals, doctors, pharmaceutical companies, and device and product manufacturers. Between 1998 and 2011, pharmaceutical companies and makers of health products spent $2.3 billion on lobbying, making them the single biggest influencer of members of Congress, who in turn pressure Medicare and federal agencies to create regulations that conform to lobbyists' interests, sometimes to the detriment of patients.

The unrecognized power of this lobby has ensured that things stay pretty much as they are in Medicare, with a reimbursement structure that rewards the most powerful players in medicine and starves hands-on therapies and primary care. That is the major unspoken reason that the 2012 health care reform bill provided for the establishment of an expert commission insulated from Congress to make many Medicare decisions, a plan that political opponents attacked as putting the fate of the elderly into the hands of "faceless bureaucrats"—rather than with the corporate and commercial lobbies and their allies in Congress, where it effectively rests now.

Anyone who attempts to open a public conversation about rehumanizing modern death must be prepared to weather charges of medical rationing, promoting "death panels," canonizing Dr. Kevorkian, and discriminating against the aged, demented, or disabled. The word "rationing" avoids the reality that our current way of dying maximizes both cost and suffering. The phrase "death panels" glosses over the fact that the mortality rate remains at 100 percent. Vilifying Dr. Kevorkian ignores the problem that many saw him as solving: the loss of autonomy near the end of life to medical overdoing. Charges of discrimination cannot mask the reality that many people consider dementia a worse fate than death; it is the demented with no close relatives who are most likely to be subjected to feeding tubes and other life-prolonging and suffering-prolonging measures. It is not age discrimination to acknowledge the reality that eighty-year-old bodies and brains don't bounce back the way young ones do, or that in the end even marathoners' bodies crumble in seven thousand irreversible ways, no matter how much technology is deployed.

One sign of the growing power of a grassroots Slow Medicine lobby can be found in New York state, where a bill promoted by Compassion and Choices and passed overwhelmingly in 2011 over strong opposition from the American Medical Association, now requires doctors to provide honest information and counseling to terminally ill patients about palliative care and hospice. But until we join most of the rest of the developed world in a universal, non-profit-driven health care system, it will remain extraordinarily difficult to follow the pathway to a Good Death, whether for yourself or for someone you love and have become responsible for.

Of course we don't want to die. We don't want to say good-bye to those we love. We certainly don't want to be the one who says to a doctor, "Enough." In this we are not alone. Our ancestors did not want to die any more than we do. Sixteenth-century lithographs show Death as a grinning skeleton who grabs a wrist and insists on dancing with farmers, apprentices, matrons, and business-men, all of them protesting that they have much more important things to do than die. But sooner or later, dance we must.

Things go better if we practice the steps of the dance before-hand. Perhaps if we find ways to make the pathway to natural death sacred and familiar again, we will recover the courage to face our deaths. If we don't, technological medicine at the end of life will continue to collude with our fear and ignorance and profit from it. Unless we create new rites of passage to help pre-pare for death long before it comes, we will remain vulnerable to the commercial exploitation of our fears and to the implied promise that death can forever be postponed.

Dying is a sacred act. Even in the worst of circumstances, it can be made holy. I know a young palliative care physician who honored a nursing-home resident who died peacefully on her unit by gathering her staff around his bed and reading a Mary Oliver poem aloud over him—a secular blessing and an honorable good-bye for a man who died without kin. I know a former pediatric oncology nurse who would take parents aside during a child's pro-tracted and painful dying and tell them they needed to let the child know that it was okay to die. After the parents' good-byes were said, the nurse told me, the child would often die peacefully, the family having been given a healing and unbillable gift, a throwback to a time when nurses were called "sister" and nursing was a religious vocation as well as a profession. Even many of the least formally religious yearn intuitively to be at peace with those they love and to resolve what remains unresolved.

It is time to honor the compassionate impulses of doctors and nurses who labor within time pressures and administrative structures that militate against accepting, discussing, and honoring dying. It is unlikely we will ever again see most deaths taking place inside the home. So we may as well admit that intensive care units and medical floors are, like it or not, hospices as well as places of lifesaving. The conference rooms where families are asked to assent to removal of life support are locations of a sacred passage and a ritual of letting-go. They should be as beautiful as those near labor and delivery rooms, with quilts on the walls, rocking chairs, and bulletin boards full of the photos of elderly people who have died on the unit, the way obstetricians often put up photographs of babies. They should not be places where the remnants of staff lunches are left, or schedules posted on walls. Even in our secular and multireligious culture, we could show our caring for these traumatized families with framed poems, or photographs of the cosmos or a lotus blossom, or any other nonspecific aspect of the sacred.

The ideal of the Good Death, as our ancestors defined it, was a natural death free of medical flailing. It did not require experts. It took place at home and was neither sudden nor lingering. Just as we do now, our ancestors hoped to die in a familiar place among close friends and family; to be safe and gently cared for in their hour of need; to have their last words heard and treasured; to express their love and forgiveness and to hear that they were loved and forgiven in turn. The impulse for the Good Death may be bred into our bones: it was once so strong that soldiers on Civil War battlefields did their best to re-create it symbolically, propping photographs of their mothers or sisters on their chests as they died far from home.

The religious among our ancestors, and there were many, used their dying moments to express their faith in God and their acceptance of His will, to repent of their sins, and to prepare their minds and souls for heaven. In the days before widespread use of effective pain medicine, the Good Death was not necessarily painless or peaceful. Our ancestors spoke of the "death agony" and the "death throes" for a reason. But it was an honest death. Nobody pretended that death was not in the room.

A brave death, to our ancestors, was one of acceptance. Today, as a glance at any day's obituaries will show, we are divided between those who "died peacefully, surrounded by family," and those honored for never giving up "the brave fight against cancer," fighting death in all its guises, and for never letting go.

My mother's death showed me another kind of courage, as I hope it has shown you. It will teach me for the rest of my life.

CHAPTER 19

A MAP THROUGH
THE LABYRINTH

What I wish I'd known:

The natural death is no longer the default pathway. If you want it for yourself or for someone you love, it is up to you to seek it out, and it is harder to find than you may think. It is not enough to sign all the right papers or to tell your friends you never want to be plugged into machines, because important decisions must be made long before your gurney is brought to the door of the emergency room after a panicked call to 911. Every mile on the way to a bad death, every "yes" to a doctor for a last-ditch treatment, every dishonest hope, may look at the time like an expression of your love and caring.

The default pathway to a disempowered death is a wide freeway with smooth, well-lit on-ramps and misleading signage about the final destination. Over time, the cars on that freeway move faster and the off-ramps grow fewer, and you may find yourself funneled toward a single stopping point, a never-say-die death in intensive care. There, at the very last moment, unfamiliar doctors may off-load onto your relatives the crushing moral burden of assenting to the discontinuance of life support.

The pathway to a natural death, on the other hand, is not so easily found. The gate may be overgrown. You will have to use your own moral compass to find it, guided by your guts, your love, and whatever support group you can scrape together. You will have to face your fears and let go of denial and hope. That is what it takes to give yourself or someone you love a chance at the kind of death our ancestors held in high esteem. You may feel alone, but you will not be alone.

The Slow Medicine path to death is a path of acceptance. It does not promise freedom from suffering. Its sufferings are plainly visible. You will need to find your way to the path of acceptance far sooner than you think, perhaps years before the actual death takes place. This is what I learned in the course of my parents' long journey through the valley of the shadow of death.

Shepherding your parents from independence to dependence and from contemplating death to dying itself may take years. It is a spiritual ordeal. Start looking for the path of acceptance at the first body blow, the day you first recognize that your parent will die someday. It could be the first stroke, or the first fall, or the first severe diabetic complication, or a diagnosis of an unambiguously fatal disease such as kidney failure, emphysema, or pancreatic or metastasized cancer. It could be the day that your mother or father loses the way home or forgets to turn off a burner and melts a pot on the stove. Your parent has entered the last stage of life. The illusion of temporary immortality is over. You cannot control whether he or she will die, but you can influence the manner of passing.

This is where the work starts. Not later. The work of death does not start on the day that someone says to you, "Your mother is dying." No one may ever say this. There may always be another treatment.

Acceptance starts with opening your heart to the reality that someone you love is approaching the end of his or her life. In whatever form speaks to you, be it poetry, letters, songs, or prayer, bring in the traditional, the holy, the beautiful. Have a birthday party for your elderly friend and say what is in your heart rather than saving it for the eulogy. Ask for a letter from your parent describing the spiritual legacy he or she would like to pass on to you. Remind yourself that this rite of passage is part of the human condition and has been traversed by others before you. It is time to find ways to say, "I love you. Thank you. Please forgive me. I forgive you." Write a legacy letter like the ones I wrote my father, naming all he had done for me. You can do all this even if your parent refuses to discuss the coming of death.

That way, when the time comes to say, "Good-bye"—and that day may come more quickly than you imagined, or it may come more slowly and require many thoughtful decisions along the way—you are ready for that, too. You may not be able to fix your parents' suffering or make them whole, but you can heal your relationships and help prepare everyone for death.

If you have said your good-byes, you will have a clearer mind and heart for the hardest decisions you have ever made, and the loneliest. In our striving secular culture, love has long been defined as giving more—more presents, faster cars, more medical fixes. The time may come when the most loving thing is to actively advocate for doing less.

CHAPTER 20

NOTES FOR
A NEW ART OF DYING

Shepherding a parent, spouse, or friend through the last phase of life encompasses six distinct, sometimes looping, stages: fragility, decline, disability, failing health, active dying, and bereavement, each one a rite of passage with its own physical and emotional tasks. These tasks include reducing expectations of medicine; maximizing independence and postponing disability; coping practically and emotionally with dependence; preparing for death; attending at the deathbed; and mourning.

Below are some notes on each stage.

STAGE 1: FRAGILITY

The older and more fragile your parent gets and the more life-threatening conditions he or she accumulates, the more critically you should look at any proposed treatment requiring general anesthesia or a hospital stay. Hospitals are dangerous places, even for the young and vigorous.

The nature of medical advocacy changes. Less is more. Discernment is the catchword.

Respect the law of diminishing returns. With each year over the age of eighty and each step down from independent functioning, physical resilience lessens, the chances of benefits dwindle, and the risks of bad medical outcomes rise. It may be preferable to live with physical limitations rather than risk mental incompetence: hip replacement, open-heart surgery, and general anesthesia all carry serious risks of cognitive decline. The time comes when an aged person will consistently come back from the hospital worse rather than better.

Shift your hopes from unrealistic "curing" to "caring," which is always possible. Maximize comfort, happiness, mobility, and independence without extending life. A hernia surgery performed under local anesthetic or stenting to relieve heart pain may be a good idea if it reduces suffering. A defibrillator or a heart bypass may extend life without improving its quality. Consider any medical treatment of an elderly person, no matter how seemingly minor, as a serious decision. Learn to tell a doctor, "No," or "Let's wait." Weigh benefits versus burdens and risks. Ask about pros, cons, and alternatives. Forget diagnostic tests such as mammograms if the results won't change plans for future treatment or nontreatment. There is no need for your parent's final years to be consumed with pointless, tiring medical appointments.

STAGE 2: DECLINE

Accepting that someone you love is beyond the reach of curative medicine is not the same as advocating medical neglect. Postpone disability, not death. Bring an occupational therapist into the home and pay out of pocket if you must: little things can be huge in preserving independence, such as balance training to prevent falls and falls training to prevent injury, as well as continence training, speech therapy, support groups, adaptive yoga, mentally stimulating day programs, and regular exercise. People with dementia who are happy and well socialized function better for longer than do the lonely and depressed. Install grab bars and take up loose rugs. I will say this although I know I am whistling in the wind: ask for and provide help *before* it's needed, not when you or your parent is on the verge of collapse. Get siblings and neighbors involved sooner rather than later. Postpone loss of independence with judicious help: a high school student hired to do driving and grocery shopping may extend the period in which a parent can remain at home and close to friends.

STAGE 3: DISABILITY

When someone can no longer function without help, family hierarchies turn upside down. Hiring independent home health aides can be cheaper than moving the parent into an assisted living complex or hiring an agency, but they take more time to manage. Research assisted living and "life care" communities carefully: sometimes the prettiest are not the best run, and this is a hard decision to undo. In her memoir and caregiving manual, *Bittersweet Season,* former *New York Times* reporter Jane Gross argues against a move to "assisted living" unless the complex also provides an excellent skilled nursing division. Think carefully before moving a parent into your home, or moving in with him or her, if your relationship has been difficult due to a parent's narcissism, violence, or substance abuse. This is where that cherished baby-boom word "boundaries" comes into play.

Caring for the Caregiver

Throughout this journey, remember you are engaged in a marathon, not a sprint. Long-term caregivers struggle with exhaustion, the grief of ambiguous loss, anger, money problems, and guilt. They are vulnerable to insomnia, depression, anxiety, neck and back pain, illness, and premature death. The typical pattern is to push to the point of collapse before gasping for help. Think in terms of two-way compassion: for the afflicted person, and for yourself.

Swallow your pride. I wish I had. The sooner you ask for help, the more you will get. Convene regular meetings or conference calls with siblings, make lists of what needs doing, and delegate. My brother Michael often lent my mother an empathic listening ear. I did medical planning, advocacy, hands-on social work, and support. Jonathan covered logistics and human resources, negotiating with Toni during the inevitable rough patches and helping my mother buy a new car. Those living far away may contribute money, while those nearby do more hands-on care.

Sometimes one adult child sacrifices a decade or more of time and earnings to caring for a parent and then receives the same inheritance as siblings who did nothing but kibitz from afar. In other cases, one sibling (usually one who isn't actively caretaking) may secretly pressure an aging parent for money or simply remove it from the bank account.

Figure out who the caregivers are and who is the support team. Give control of money and decisions to whoever is doing the bulk of the hands-on work. Don't let brothers off the hook; I wish I'd been more direct with mine. If there is money available, consider openly paying the sibling who carries most of the burden or giving that sibling a larger portion of the estate. Better to handle this aboveboard than let resentments fester long after death.

Ambivalence is part of the job. Vent to a friend, partner, therapist, social-media group, or support group.

Clarify limits. Strive for imperfection. Do what you can when you can, and say no when you must. It's better to do a little consistently than go overboard and then withdraw. Local members of the National Association of Area Agencies on Aging (www.n4a.org) offer respite services for lower-income families.

STAGE 4: FAILING HEALTH

A parent may go through months or even years of "failing," perhaps becoming bedridden, before entering the three-to-ten-day process that hospice workers call "active dying." Listen to what your parents say and also what is left unsaid. When someone says, "No more hospitals," or "I'm living too long," consider this an invitation to unpack the implications of the statement. Does this mean he would rather die than go through another hospitalization or enter a nursing home? On what terms do they consider their lives worth living? Do the emotional work of preparing for death even though it may be months away. Some hospice programs offer workshops in "anticipatory loss," and you can pay out of pocket if the one you love is not enrolled yet as a hospice patient. Consider a palliative care program and discuss the legal papers discussed at length below.

Palliative care is not a death-oriented practice. It is devoted to maximizing quality of life and comfort while living with chronic illness, including but not limited to conditions that are life threatening and ultimately fatal. For people with serious illnesses in their last years (as opposed to months) of life, it provides many of the benefits of hospice, including a practical team that visits the home and focuses on maximizing function and controlling symptoms. Many hospitals now have inpatient palliative-care departments. Outpatient (visiting-nurse-style) palliative programs are becoming popular. If you don't ask, you may not get: the doctor assigned to your case in the hospital may or may not choose to refer you to palliative care, depending on his or her personal medical philosophy. Except in New York state, the doctor has no ethical or legal obligation to do so. So speak up. In my experience, both doctors and family members tend to overestimate how much time a family member has before death knocks at the door.

Admittance to a palliative care program does not require a doctor's letter that death is on the horizon, nor does it require forgoing curative treatments. But a palliative care patient can segue smoothly into hospice care, because the philosophy—comfort first, shared decision making, clarity about medical goals, coordinated support for the whole family, pragmatism, and limiting burdensome interventions—is similar. (Hospice is a type of palliative care, and both are forms of Slow Medicine, but not all palliative care is hospice.) Palliative care can sometimes prolong life better than more aggressive medicine. A study reported in 2010 in the *New England Journal of Medicine* found that lung cancer patients receiving early palliative care were hospitalized less frequently and declined more invasive treatments. They also experienced less depression and increased quality of life, and survived 2.7 months longer than those receiving standard oncological care.

If you sense that your parent or spouse is on the final downward slide, advocate forcefully for admittance to hospice or palliative care sooner rather than later. To qualify for hospice care, you must find a sympathetic physician willing to sign a letter saying that the patient is expected to die within six months, will forgo all curative treatments, and will accept only symptom management, pain control, and "comfort care." (You can, however, de-enroll from hospice care if you change your mind or regain your health, and reenter later.) Patients with certain cancers and other clearly life-ending diagnoses qualify most easily, but those with "the dwindles" or heart failure or dementia can qualify, too. Doctors frequently overestimate how long their patients have left: my father was approved for hospice only ten days before his death, my mother, thirty days. Your local hospice may be able to refer you to a doctor who shares your values.

STAGE 5: ACTIVE DYING

When a patient starts to die in a nursing home, it is often standard protocol to call 911 and to subject the dying person to violent CPR, even though only 3 percent of nursing-home residents (and other frail and dependent elderly people) benefit from CPR, and some survive only to die again a week later. Ask if your family member can get hospice care within the nursing home. Unfortunately, Medicare sometimes forces a choice between skilled nursing services and hospice: you can still get both services, but must pay out of pocket for one. A do-not-resuscitate order reinforced by a state-recognized bracelet, as discussed below, is often an act of realism and mercy.

A "do not hospitalize" order can also be a mercy, because it is standard protocol in many nursing homes to move a dying patient to the hospital, sometimes resulting in repeated bouncing back and forth (known in hospital argot as "turfing") in the last few months of life. The reasons have little to do with the peace and comfort of the patient and a great deal to do with the economics of our Kafkaesque reimbursement system and institutional fears of legal liability. Physician's Orders for Life-Sustaining Treatment (POLST) signed by a doctor can reduce the risk, as explained below. Again, being enrolled in hospice or palliative care reduces the chance of terminal manhandling, because the nursing home no longer has to worry about being sued for medical neglect by a Nephew from Peoria.

Hospice programs provide teams of visiting nurses, social

workers, and volunteers, and other forms of familial and patient support. Due to a slow erosion in financial reimbursements, however, they no longer provide enough hands-on nursing care to keep a patient comfortable without supplementation from a full-time family caregiver or hired aides.

A word about dementia: it is a terminal illness and often a miserable death. Don't draw it out. Feeding tubes are uncomfortable, and stopping eating and drinking are natural, painless, traditional gateways to death. (Many alert old people with incurable illnesses voluntarily stop eating and drinking, one of the few methods legally and practically open to them for ending their lives.) The pain of infections can be managed with painkillers rather than antibiotics. Depriving a demented parent of a natural death may seem loving, but it is rarely kind. Think about whether your actions are bringing more or less suffering to your parent and to the world. Comfort yourself: it is the demented with no family who are most likely to be subjected to feeding tubes and antibiotics in their last weeks and months of life. Saying no is often an expression of love.

Dying is not an emergency. Emergency rooms, 911 systems, and intensive care units are all primed to prevent natural death. Engage with them with caution. The most important sentences in this book may be, "I request a palliative care consult," "Can you refer me to hospice?" "I request comfort measures only," and "I am concerned about quality of life."

STAGE 6: BEREAVEMENT

Once upon a time, when people were more likely to be born and to die in the same town, grieving and mourning were community events, not psychological diagnoses. In Victorian times, widows wore black for at least a year, and sometimes for life.

For decades after the carnage of World War I, British people in villages, towns, and cities lined up on the streets once a year to observe a shared five minutes of memorial silence.

In my childhood in England, amid the ruined buildings left by the German bombardment of the Second World War, people tied black bands around their jacket sleeves and wore them all through the day when they attended funerals. Mourning was not an embarrassment in those days, not so long ago. When I was in my twenties and living in San Francisco's North Beach, I'd watch brass bands parade slowly down Green Street in front of Chinese funeral processions, the black hearses decked with flowers and photographs. I can't help thinking that if we spoke of death more directly and honored its sacredness more—rather than honoring only "the sacredness of life" and pretending that death isn't part of Nature or God's plan—we might respond more wisely in its face, and more fully afterward.

There is less permission to grieve and mourn openly today, and it's especially hard for those who live far away from parents and birthplaces. The ones who love us best don't necessarily know our parents; those who loved our parents often barely know us. And yet, at the great turning points—as we cross the thresholds of birth, marriage, adulthood, and the final, inevitable loss of our earthly personality and all we love—we often hunger for ritual and community.

Let the funeral or memorial service bless you with the healing power of shared grieving. Fall into the old forms, remake them as you need to, and let them support you. Don't be tyrannized by the notion of "closure," or be too quick to call the service a "celebration of life," or to tell those who gather not to shed tears. Rituals—particularly holding my parents' memorial services, responding to condolence letters, and lighting Yahrzeit candles each year in remembrance of them—helped me give form to the deep, complicated emotions (sorrow, regret, agony, numbness, loss, guilt, exhaustion, remorse, a hunger for solitude, irritability, and secret relief) that I felt after they died.

Most people I know who've helped their parents through the final passage regret having done too much or too little, or are haunted by their parents' suffering during deaths that came too soon or too late. Please forgive yourself. You've done your best. Do not be tyrannized by the notion of the Good Death.

Hospice programs offer bereavement groups, and some county mental health associations offer grief counseling. If you do not qualify for free services, you can usually pay modestly out of pocket. I found the program at my local hospice excellent, and well worth what I paid.

RESOURCES

I found the following books and resources helpful.

Caregiving and Medical Advocacy

Bailey, Elizabeth. *The Patient's Checklist.* New York: Sterling, 2011. A sobering, defensive manual for reducing the risks attending hospital stays.

Byock, Ira. *Dying Well: Peace and Possibilities at the End of Life.* New York: Riverhead Books, 1997. A beautiful guide to the emotional work at the approach of the end of life.

Coste, Joanne Koenig. *Learning to Speak Alzheimer's: A Groundbreaking Approach for Everyone Dealing with the Disease.* New York: Houghton Mifflin, 2003.

Dunn, Hank. *Hard Choices for Loving People.* Lansdowne, VA: A & A Publishers, 2009. Written by a hospice chaplain, this simple eighty-page pamphlet is worth its weight in gold. A moral and practical framework for medical decisions, with sections on palliative care, CPR, feeding tubes, antibiotics, respirators, dialysis, and intravenous fluids.

Gross, Jane. *A Bittersweet Season: Caring for Our Aging Parents—and Ourselves.* New York: Alfred A. Knopf, 2011. Guidance on Medicare, Medicaid, nursing homes, and assisted living. Gross has also prepared "Caring for the Elderly" (http://www.nytimes.com/ref/health/noa_resources.html), an exhaustive resource guide from the *New York Times's* excellent "New Old Age" blog, which Gross pioneered. http://newoldage.blogs.nytimes.com.

McCullough, Dennis. *My Mother, Your Mother: Embracing "Slow Medicine,"*

The Compassionate Approach to Caring for Your Aging Loved Ones. New York: HarperCollins, 2007. The single best manual on medical caregiving in the years stretching from decline to death, by a leading geriatrician formerly of Dartmouth Medical School.

Moyers, Bill. "On Our Own Terms." Four-part *Frontline* series on end-of-life care in America, available on DVD at libraries and on Netflix.

Caring for the Caregiver

Boss, Pauline. *Ambiguous Loss: Learning to Live with Unresolved Grief*. Cambridge, MA: Harvard University Press, 1999.

Hargrave, Terry. *Loving Your Parents When They Can No Longer Love You*. Grand Rapids, MI: Zondervan, 2005. Excellent guide to familial caregiving issues, from the perspective of a Christian psychotherapist.

Jacobs, Barry. *The Emotional Survival Guide for Caregivers*. New York: Guildford Press, 2006.

Kabat-Zinn, Jon. *Full Catastrophe Living*. New York: Delacorte Press, 1990.

Lao-tzu. *Tao Te Ching*. Translated by Stephen Mitchell. New York: Harper & Row, 1988.

Satow, Roberta. *Doing the Right Thing: Taking Care of Your Elderly Parents Even if They Didn't Take Care of You*. New York: Penguin, 1995. Another excellent guide to familial caregiving issues, from the perspective of a New York psychoanalyst.

Government Support

The federal Family and Medical Leave Act guarantees family caregivers *unpaid* time off from work without risking job termination. California and New Jersey go a step further and provide several weeks per year of "paid family leave," akin to unemployment insurance payments, to payroll workers who miss work to care for a sick parent or other relative. Washington State has a similar program, but it is restricted to those caring for children. The District of Columbia requires employers to provide some paid family leave. California's program, administered through its Employment Development Department, is the most generous: family caregivers can be compensated for up to six weeks per year. Work absences don't have to be consecutive, and the program covers caregiving performed in another state or done over the phone.

In most states, elderly people poor enough to qualify for Medicaid can pay their family caregivers through the National Resource Center for Participant-Directed Services. See "How to Get Financial Help for Taking Care of Mom, Dad" at AARP.org's Caregiving Resource Center. http://www.AARP.org/relation ships/caregiving-resource-center.

Organizations

The American Association of Retired Persons (AARP) has excellent tips and articles in its Caregiving Resource Center under the "Home and Family" tab on its Web site, http://www.AARP.org.

Your local Alzheimer's Association, listed in the white pages, offers support groups for families coping with all forms of dementia. http://www.alz.org. 1-800-272-3900.

The Family Caregiver Alliance offers classes and legislative advocacy for a huge, neglected interest group. http://www.caregiver.org. 785 Market Street, Suite 750, San Francisco, CA 94103. 415-434-3388; 1-800-445-8106.

The Center to Advance Palliative Care (CAPC) has an excellent, user-friendly Web site for families that explains palliative care and lists programs by city and state. http://www.getpalliativecare.org. 1255 Fifth Avenue, Suite C-2, New York, NY 10029. 1-212-201-2670.

The National Hospice and Palliative Care Organization can refer you to local hospice providers, and its Web site features guides to palliative care, Medicare coverage, and how to open a discussion of end-of-life wishes. http://www.nhpco .org. 1731 King Street, Suite 100, Alexandria, Virginia 22314. 1-800-658-8898.

Compassion and Choices, which advocates for right-to-die laws and the legalization of physician-assisted suicide, provides free counseling for families seeking to withdraw or refuse medical treatment and facing institutional resistance. We used their service, and found it helpful. http://www.compassionand choices.org. P.O Box 101810, Denver, CO 80250. 1-800-247-7421.

General Readings

For an overview of the death-ways we've lost, and where that loss has taken us, I recommend:

Aries, Philippe. *Western Attitudes toward Death from the Middle Ages to the Present*. Baltimore: John Hopkins University Press, 1974.
Brownlee, Shannon. *Overtreatment: Why Too Much Medicine Is Making Us Sicker and Poorer*. New York: Bloomsbury, 2007.
Nuland, Sherwin B. *How We Die: Reflections on Life's Final Chapter*. New York: Vintage Books, 1993.

LEGALITIES

You have a constitutional right to refuse any medical treatment or ask for its withdrawal on your own behalf or on behalf of someone who has legally entrusted you with that role. Some family members have even called an ambulance and signed someone out of an intensive care unit against medical advice. Your right to medical autonomy trumps any doctor's conception of his or her Hippocratic oath to act with beneficence, which doctors may wrongfully interpret as meaning that they should always do more (and that you should go along). If a doctor is unwilling to do as you ask, he or she is obligated to refer you to someone who will. If you and the doctor aren't on the same page, find another. Any request on behalf of incommunicado patients should legally be phrased in terms of your understanding of their wishes, not your own sense of what is best for them. (You may be guided by their "best interests" only if their wishes are not known.)

Having your paperwork in order is often promoted as the be-all and end-all of a good death. Unfortunately, it's not that simple. But it is a start.

Do Not Resuscitate

Signed by both patient and doctor, a DNR affirms your right to a natural death free of electrical defibrillation and chest pounding. Given the dismal survival rates of those resuscitated outside hospitals, it isn't as radical as it sounds. If you call 911 in a panic, however, emergency medical technicians *will* resuscitate you or your family member, even if you have a DNR, unless you have further, state-approved DNR identification, usually an official plastic bracelet. Regulations vary by state, but all recognize a metal bracelet purchasable from the Medic-Alert Foundation. http://www.medicalert.org. 1-888-633-4298.

Advance Directives ("Living Wills")

Better than nothing, the outdated, boilerplate versions of these documents offered by many lawyers ask for no life support only when you are comatose or within six months of death. For a tailored document that includes more specific instructions on gray-area issues such as dementia, antibiotics, feeding tubes, and devices like pacemakers, see an elder lawyer or a doctor specializing in palliative care or geriatrics. One such nationally known specialist is Jennifer Brokaw, MD, at the group medical practice Good Medicine in San Francisco, CA.

Physician's Orders for Life-Sustaining Treatment (POLST)

Signed by both physician and patient, and printed on bright-pink attention-getting paper, POLST orders carry more weight with doctors and hospitals than living wills and DNRs. They are more specific and cover respirators, unnecessary transfers and hospitalizations, feeding tubes, antibiotics, and intravenous fluids. They have a box to check for "comfort measures only."

POLST California has a downloadable version. http://www.capolst.org.

The Coalition for Compassionate Care of California has an excellent guide to legal-medical paperwork. http://www.coalitionccc.org/advance-health-plan ning.php.

For a clear, quick introduction to advance planning, see the *San Jose Mercury News*'s excellent "Cost of Dying" pages by Lisa Krieger. http://www.mercu rynews.com/cost-of-dying.

Medical Guardianship

A Durable Power of Attorney for Health Care gives someone you trust the authority to make your medical choices when you can no longer make your own. Like the other legal documents, this is only a start, and not a substitute for expressing your wishes and getting agreement in careful family meetings. Unless all family members are on the same page, doctors often override the "health care proxy" and provide maximum treatment due to fear of litigation.

WHEN COMMUNICATION BREAKS DOWN

Hospitals are worlds unto themselves, with fragmented, tribalistic, and often nonexistent chains of command. Essentially they provide operating rooms, nursing, and diagnostic services, while each doctor uses the facility and bills separately as an independent contractor. If auto-repair shops were organized like hospitals, you would get one bill from the mechanic who fixed the radiator, another from the guy who did the brakes and fixed the sunroof, and yet another from the one who provided the shop floor and the lift. Each would focus on his own specialty, and nobody would supervise anyone else.

The result is often fragmentation of care and too many cooks, each narrowly focused on repairing a single vital organ, with no overall plan. A palliative care physician can help provide a coherent plan. A patient liaison, hospital social worker, hospice physician, hospitalist, or staff bioethicist can also help you negotiate this confusing culture. If your relative is getting too much, too little, or the wrong kind of care, ask for a bioethics or palliative care consult. Some hospitals have anonymous bioethics hotlines.

PACEMAKERS AND DEFIBRILLATORS: YOUR LEGAL AND MORAL RIGHT TO DEACTIVATION

Experts appointed by the American Heart Association, the Heart Rhythm Society, and the American College of Cardiologists have stated that disabling a pacemaker or defibrillator is neither assisted suicide nor euthanasia. Refer your physician to:

Lampert, Rachel, et al. "HRS Expert Consensus Statement on the Management of Cardiovascular Implantable Electronic Devices (CIEDs) in Patients Nearing the End of Life or Requesting Withdrawal of Therapy." *Heart Rhythm.* 7, no. 7 (July, 2010): 1008–1026. Available from the Heart Rhythm Society online under the section "Clinical Guidelines and Documents." http://www.hrsonline.org/Practice-Guidance/Clinical-Guidelines-Documents/Expert-Consensus-Statement-on-the-Management-of-CIEDs.

BAD DEATHS

These cautionary tales show what is in store for the unprepared:

Krieger, Lisa. "The Cost of Dying: It's Hard to Reject Care Even as Costs Soar." *San Jose Mercury News,* Feb. 5, 2012. http://www.mercurynews.com/cost-of-dying/ci_19898736. A blow-by-blow account of her eighty-eight-year-old father's ten-day, $323,000 death in an intensive care unit.

Windrum, Bart. *Notes from the Waiting Room: How to Survive a Parent's End-of-Life Hospitalization.* Boulder, CO: Axiom Action, 2008. This confusingly organized book contains valuable practical advice starting on page 60.

Wolff, Michael. "A Life Worth Ending: The Era of Medical Miracles Has Created a New Phase of Aging, as Far from Living as It Is from Dying. A Son's Plea to Let His Mother Go." *New York,* May 20, 2012. http://nymag.com/news/features/parent-health-care-2012–5. Heart-valve surgery fixed his mother's heart and worsened her dementia.

BEREAVEMENT

Hospice programs provide free bereavement groups and counseling to family members of their patients for a full year after death. Others can pay out of pocket, often on a sliding scale. See also:

Safer, Jeanne. *Death Benefits: How Losing a Parent Can Change an Adult's Life—for the Better.* New York: Basic Books, 2010.

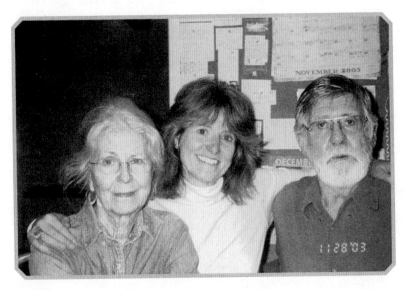

Valerie, Katy, and Jeffrey Butler, Pine Street, Middletown, Connecticut, November 2003.

NOTES

vii *Epigraph*: "I Fell," by Makeda, Queen of Sheba, translated by Jane Hirshfield, from Jane Hirshfield, ed., *Women in Praise of the Sacred.* (New York: HarperCollins, 1994).

PROLOGUE

3 *Whenever there is someone in a family*: Anton Chekhov, *Peasants and Other Stories* (New York: New York Review of Books, 1999), 328. From the short story "Peasants."

4 *a doctor might well feel duty-bound*: More than half of demented nursing home residents receive antibiotics in their last two weeks of life. Erika D'Agata and Susan L. Mitchell, "Patterns of Antimicrobial Use among Nursing Home Residents with Advanced Dementia," *Archives of Internal Medicine* 168, no. 4 (2008): 357–62.

4 *Three-quarters of Americans want to die at home*: See, for example, Lake Research Partners and the Coalition for Compassionate Care of California, *Final Chapter: Californians' Attitudes and Experiences with Death and Dying* (Oakland: California Health Care Foundation, 2012), 1, accessed

September 23, 2012, http://www.chcf.org/publications/2012/02/final-chapter-death-dying.

4 *Two-fifths of deaths*: "Underlying Cause of Death 1999–2009 on CDC WONDER Online Database," Centers for Disease Control and Prevention, National Center for Health Statistics, released 2012.

5 *a fifth of American deaths now take place in intensive care*: Allan Garland, "Improving the Intensive Care Unit," in *Surgical Intensive Care Medicine*, 2nd ed., ed. John M. O'Donnell and Flávio E. Nácul (New York: Springer, 2009), 685.

5 *can cost as much as $323,000*: Lisa Krieger, "The Cost of Dying," *San Jose Mercury News*, February 5, 2012, accessed September 23, 2012, http://www.mercurynews.com/cost-of-dying/ci_19898736.

6 *like an armed man*: the phrase is from Daniel Defoe's semifictional account of the Great Plague of London, *A Journal of the Plague Year* (London, 1722).

7 *a quarter of Medicare's roughly $560 billion*: Gerald F. Riley and James D. Lubitz, "Long-Term Trends in Medicare Payments in the Last Year of Life," *Health Services Research* 45, no. 2 (2010): 565–76; and "Medicare," Congressional Budget Office, accessed August 16, 2012, http://www.cbo.gov/topics/retirement/medicare.

1: ALONG CAME A BLACKBIRD

14 *It is a predictable hazard*: Sherwin B. Nuland, *How We Die: Reflections on Life's Final Chapter* (New York: Knopf, 1994), 65.

20 *He thanked Sir Alexander Fleming*: Richard Tames, *Penicillin: A Breakthrough in Medicine* (Chicago: Reed Elsevier, 2000), 20.

26 *prolonged and attenuated dying*: this beautiful phrase was coined by the pioneering geriatrician Dennis McCullough, author of *My Mother, Your Mother: Embracing "Slow Medicine," the Compassionate Approach to Caring for Your Aging Loved Ones* (New York: HarperCollins, 2008). I thank him for permission to use it here.

2: A YEAR OF GRACE

32 *one of twenty-nine million unpaid*: National Alliance for Caregiving and AARP, *Caregiving in the U.S. 2009* (Bethesda, MD: NAC and AARP, 2009).

33 *The requirements are so draconian*: Medicare Payment Advisory Commission, "Report to the Congress: Medicare Payment Policy (March 2012)," 282, http://www.medpac.gov/chapters/Mar12_Ch11.pdf.

34 *I discovered that the entry for Ambien*: Paul Walsh, ed., PDR 56 Edition 2002 *Physicians' Desk Reference* (Montvale, NJ: Medical Economics/ Thomson Healthcare, 2002), 3194.

35 *nearly twenty-four million sons and daughters*: National Alliance for Caregiving and AARP, *Caregiving in the U.S. 2009* (Bethesda: NAC and AARP, 2009). This describes a slightly different statistical cohort from the one on p. 34.

35 *Some European countries*: Mark Merlis, "Caring for the Frail Elderly: An International Review," *Health Affairs* 19, no. 3 (2000): 141–49.

35 *Not in the United States*: The limited exceptions are a few state programs and federal payments to family members caring for impoverished Medicaid patients, discussed in more detail in "Resources."

35 *But even though our parents*: June R. Lunney, Joanne Lynn, and Christopher Hogan, "Profiles of Older Medicare Decedents," *Journal of the American Geriatrics Society* 50, no. 6 (2002): 1108–112.

36 *37 percent of baby-boom women*: I-Fen Lin and Susan L. Brown, "Unmarried Boomers Confront Old Age: A National Portrait," *Gerontologist* 52, no. 2 (2012): 153–65.

38 *Medicare funds mainly one-to-one interactions*: Public Affairs Specialist Ellen Griffith, Centers for Medicare and Medicaid Services, e-mail message to author, May 2, 2012.

3: RITES OF PASSAGE

47 *just as it covers 45 percent*: Senate Special Committee on Aging, *Long-Term Care Report,* 107th Cong., 2d sess., 2002, S. Prt. 107–74.

4: THE TYRANNY OF HOPE

57 *By the age of seventy-five*: Sherwin B. Nuland, *How We Die: Reflections on Life's Final Chapter* (New York: Knopf, 1994), 53.

58 *Slow Medicine*: Alberto Dolara, "Invitation to 'Slow Medicine,'" *Italian Heart Journal Supplement* 3, no. 1 (2002): 100–101.

58 *Excessive eagerness to act*: Alberto Dolara, "Avoiding Haste in Clinical Cardiology," *Acta Cardiologica* 60, no. 6 (2005): 569–73.

59 *To do more . . . is not necessarily to do better*: Interview with Francesco Fiorista, April 2012. See also Francesco Fiorista, "'Fast Medicine' and 'Slow Medicine,'" *Italian Heart Journal Supplement* 3, no. 6 (2002): 685.

59 *more likely than their doctors to reject*: Dawn Stacey, et al., "Decision Aids for People Facing Health Treatment or Screening Decisions," *Cochrane*

Database of Systematic Reviews 10 (2011): 38, doi: 10.1002/14651858 .CD001431.pub3.

59 *nearly half of patients say they don't get*: Mick P. Couper, "Medical Decisions in America: the Patient Perspective," PowerPoint presentation, Foundation for Informed Medical Decision Making Research and Policy Forum, Washington DC, January 28, 2009.

59 *30 percent of seriously ill people*: T. J. Mattimore, et al., "Surrogate and Physician Understanding of Patients' Preferences for Living Permanently in a Nursing Home," *Journal of American Geriatrics Society* 45, no. 7 (1997): 818–24.

60 *28 percent of people with congestive heart failure*: Eldrin F. Lewis, et al., "Preferences for Quality of Life or Survival Expressed by Patients with Heart Failure," *Journal of Heart and Lung Transplantation* 20, no. 9 (2001): 1016–24. See also Lynne W. Stevenson, et al., "Changing Preferences for Survival after Hospitalization with Advanced Heart Failure," *Journal of the American College of Cardiology* 5 (2008): 1702–8, doi:10.1016/jacc.2008.08.028.

63 *decried as reimbursement for "death panels"*: Jim Dwyer, "Distortions on Health Bill, Homegrown," *New York Times,* August 25, 2009, accessed May 28, 2012, http://www.nytimes.com/2009/08/26/nyregion/26about .html?ref=betsymccaugheyross.

63 *would probably not have lived*: This is an area of controversy, as nobody knows with certainty how long my father would have lived without the device. Many cardiologists argue that pacemakers improve quality of life and do not as a rule extend life. Others note that as hearts further deteriorate with age and new problems emerge, some patients become "pacemaker dependent" and are likely to die suddenly if the device is deactivated. (My father, for instance, was given diagnoses of paroxysmal atrial fibrillation and worsening heart block in the last two years of his life.) Little allowance seems to be made for a gray area, and some studies suggest increased longevity for those with pacemakers. See Ann G. Coumbe et al., "Long-term follow-up of older patients with Mobitz type I second degree atrioventricular block," *Heart,* October 19, 2012, accessed December 5, 2012, http://www.heart.bmj.com. Because of the specific case discussed in chapter 18 and others not cited, I have chosen to rely on the forecasts of my father's internist and cardiologist, both of whom believed he would have died within a year or two without a device.

64 *world's second-largest manufacturer of pacemakers*: Janet Moore, "Pacemakers: Still Ticking at Age 50," *Minneapolis Star-Tribune,* September 28, 2008, accessed May 1, 2012, http://www.startribune.com/busi ness/29828484.html.

65 *agreements that keep negotiated prices secret*: James Walsh, "Secrecy on Medical-Device Prices Hurts Buyers, GAO Says," *Minneapolis Star Tribune,* February 11, 2012. Includes an interview with Curtis Rooney, President, Healthcare Supply Chain Association.

65 *pacemaker prices*: Barry Meier, "As Their Use Soars, Heart Implants Raise
    Questions," *New York Times,* August 2, 2005, accessed May 9, 2012, http://
    www.nytimes.com/2005/08/02/business/02device.html?pagewanted=3&_
    r=1.

65 *one hospital paid $8,723 more*: Government Accountability Office,
    Medicare: Lack of Price Transparency May Hamper Hospitals' Ability to
    Be Prudent Purchasers of Implantable Medical Devices (2012), GAO-
    12–126, 26.

5: INVENTING LIFESAVING AND TRANSFORMING DEATH

For the birth of cardiac technology I relied mainly on Kirk Jeffrey, *Machines in Our Hearts: The Cardiac Pacemaker, the Implantable Defibrillator, and American Health Care* (Baltimore, MD: Johns Hopkins University Press, 2001), especially chapter 2. For Peter Bent Brigham, I drew on Renee Fox, *Experiment Perilous: Physicians and Patients Facing the Unknown* (Glencoe, IL: Free Press, 1959); Renée C. Fox and Judith P. Swazey, *The Courage to Fail: A Social View of Organ Transplants and Dialysis* (Chicago: University of Chicago Press, 1973); and Atul Gawande, "Desperate Measures," *New Yorker,* May 5, 2003, 70–81, an invaluable narrative of the "black years" at the Brigham that alerted me to Moore's subsequent suicide.

66 *The year was 1952; the place, Beth Israel Hospital in Boston*: Kirk Jef-
    frey, *Machines in Our Hearts: The Cardiac Pacemaker, the Implantable
    Defibrillator, and American Health Care* (Baltimore, MD: Johns Hopkins
    University Press, 2001), 36; P. M. Zoll, "Resuscitation of the Heart in
    Ventricular Standstill by External Electric Stimulation," *New England
    Journal of Medicine* 247 (1952): 768–71; P. M. Zoll, "Development of
    Electric Control of Cardiac Rhythm," *Journal of the American Medical
    Association* 226, no. 8 (1973): 881–86.

68 *intense repeated shocks*: David C. Schechter, "Background of Clinical
    Cardiac Electrostimulation VI: Precursor Apparatus and Events to the
    Electrical Treatment of Complete Heart Block," *New York State Journal
    of Medicine* 72 (1972): 954. Jeffrey, *Machines in Our Hearts,* 53.

68 *had been on an external Zoll pacemaker*: Interview with Seymour Fur-
    man by Earl E. Bakken, Minneapolis, MN, August 14, 1980, Pioneers
    in Pacing Video Series, Bakken Museum and Library; Seymour Furman,
    "Attempted Suicide," editorial, *Pacing and Clinical Electrophysiology* 3
    (1980): 129; quoted in Jeffrey, *Machines in Our Hearts,* 54.

70 *a young kidney doctor*: Fox and Swazey, *Courage to Fail,* 202–3; Debo-
    rah Illman, ed., "Pioneers in Kidney Dialysis: From the Scribner Shunt

and the Mini-II to the 'One-Button Machine,'" *Pathbreakers: A Century of Excellence in Science and Technology at the University of Washington* (University of Washington, 1996), accessed April 30, 2012, http://www.washington.edu/research/pathbreakers/1960c.html.

71 *hearts that stopped beating*: W. B. Kouwenhoven, et al., "Closed-Chest Cardiac Massage," *Journal of the American Medical Association* 173, no. 10 (1960): 1064–67; Diana Berry, "History of Cardiology: Desmond Julian, M.D." *Circulation,* 115(22) (2007):113–14.

71 *Some surgeons used sterilized Dacron*: Interview with Nicolas Tilney, MD, December 2011.

72 *At the Brigham in peacetime*: J. J. Collins and Dwight Harken. "The Legacy of Mitral Valvuloplasty," *Journal of Cardiac Surgery* 9 (1994): 210; cited in Nicholas Tilney, *A Perfectly Striking Departure* (Sagamore Beach, MA: Science History Publications, 2006).

72 *Six out of ten*: W. Gerald Rainer, "Pioneer Interviews: Dr. Dwight Harken," Cardiothoracic Surgery Network, July 4, 2004, http://www.ctsnet.org/sections/residents/pioneerinterviews/article-1.html. See also Stephen Westaby and Cecil Bosher, *Landmarks in Cardiac Surgery* 147 (Oxford, England: Isis Medical Media Ltd., 1997).

72 *Among those who died*: Dwight Harken, "Fifteen-to-Twenty-Year Study of One Thousand Patients Undergoing Closed Mitral Valvuloplasty," *Circulation* 48 (1973): 357–64.

72 *remove the pituitary glands from women*: Atul Gawande, "Desperate Measures," *New Yorker,* May 5, 2003, 70–81.

73 *specialist in medical ethics*: Paul Ramsey, *The Patient as Person* (New Haven, CT: Yale University Press, 1970), 238.

73 *With their new machines and new skills*: "Surgery, the Best Hope of All," *Time,* May 3, 1963, accessed December 20, 2011, special issue available at http://www.time.com.

73 *all nine Brigham patients who received experimental liver transplants*: Atul Gawande, "Desperate Measures," *New Yorker,* May 5, 2003, 70–81.

73 *The patients selected*: Francis D. Moore, *A Miracle and a Privilege: Recounting a Half Century of Surgical Advance* (Washington, DC: Joseph Henry Press, 1995), 161.

74 *would cool the child's body*: James Fogerty, *Converzatione* with Manuel Villafaña, "Pioneers of the Medical Device Industry in Minnesota Oral History Project," Minnesota Historical Society, St. Paul, Minnesota, November 20, 1997, 68.

74 *seven in a row of Lillehei's "blue babies"*: Wayne G. Miller, *King of Hearts: The True Story of the Maverick Who Pioneered Open Heart Surgery* (New York: Times Books, 2000), 62, 148.

75 *Bakken was tinkering in his family's basement*: Interview with David Rhees by Earl Bakken, "Pioneers of the Medical Device Industry in Minnesota Oral History Project," Minnesota Historical Society, Fridley, Minnesota, August 28, 1997.

76 *In the fall of 1958*: This milestone is often mistakenly attributed to Wilson Greatbatch, who invented a version of the implantable pacemaker the following year. See Jeffrey, *Machines in Our Hearts*, 96–105; and in contrast, Barnaby Feder, "Wilson Greatbatch, Inventor of Implantable Pacemaker, Dies at 92," *New York Times*, September 28, 2011, accessed September 24, 2012, http://www.nytimes.com/2011/09/28/business/wilson-greatbatch-pacemaker-inventor-dies-at-92.html.

76 *the director of research*: Janet Moore, "Pacemakers: Still Ticking at Age 50," *Minneapolis Star-Tribune*, September 28, 2008, accessed May 1, 2012, http://www.startribune.com/business/29828484.html.

77 *nation's first "crash carts"*: William Colby, *Unplugged: Reclaiming Our Right to Die in America* (New York: AMACOM, 2006), 62–66.

78 *There was no hope*: Joyce James, *Dubliners* (New York: Random House, 1954), 7.

79 *anxiety, depression, and symptoms of post-traumatic stress*: Elie Azoulay, et al., "Risk of Post-Traumatic Stress Symptoms in Family Members of Intensive Care Unit Patients," *American Journal of Respiratory and Critical Care Medicine* 171 (2005): 987–94.

79 *like spare parts*: Renée C. Fox and Judith P. Swazey, *Spare Parts: Organ Replacement in American Society* (New York: Oxford University Press, 1992).

81 *Hang in there!*: Shinmon Aoki, *Coffinman: The Journal of a Buddhist Mortician*, trans. Wayne Yokoyama (Anaheim, CA: Buddhist Education Center, 2002), 52–53.

81 *a study in the* Lancet: J. D. Hill, et al., "A Randomized Trial of Home-Versus-Hospital Management for Patients with Suspected Myocardial Infarction," *Lancet* 311, no. 8069 (1978): 837.

81 *Another study*: H. G. Mather, et al., "Myocardial Infarction: A Comparison between Home and Hospital Care for Patients," *British Medical Journal* 1, no. 6015 (1976): 928.

81 *about 2 percent of beds*: "Emergency Activity and Critical Care Capacity," U.K. Department of Health, accessed June 24, 2012, http://www.dh.gov.uk/en/Publicationsandstatistics/Statistics/Performancedataandstatistics/EmergencyActivityandCriticalCareCapacity/index.htm.

81 *in the United States*: "Health Forum, 2010 American Hospital Association Annual Survey of Hospitals," American Hospital Association. Not all respondents completed this section of the survey, so the actual proportion may be higher.

83 *This case report is submitted for publication*: William St. Clair Symmers, "Correspondence: Not Allowed to Die," *British Medical Journal* 1 (1968): 442.

84 *As he later wrote in his autobiography*: Francis D. Moore, M.D., *A Miracle and a Privilege: Recounting a Half Century of Surgical Advance* (Washington, D.C.: Joseph Henry Press, 1995), 237.

87 *The fundamental principles*: Diane E. Meier, Stephen L. Isaacs, and

Robert Hughes, *Palliative Care: Transforming the Care of Serious Illness* (San Francisco: Jossey-Bass, 2010), 24.

6: MY FATHER'S OPEN HEART

88 *somewhere between 6 and 30 percent*: Terri G. Monk and Barbara G. Phillips-Bute, "Longitudinal Assessment of Neurocognitive Function in Elderly Patients after Major, Noncardiac Surgery," *Anesthesiology* 101 (2004): A62; J. Canet, et al., "Cognitive Dysfunction after Minor Surgery in the Elderly," *Acta Anaesthesiologica Scandinavica* 47 (2003): 1204–10.

92 *In a further reflection*: Eileen Boris and Jennifer Klein, "Home-Care Workers Aren't Just 'Companions,'" *New York Times* Opinion Pages, July 1, 2012.

98 *To Any Young Soldier*: Guy Butler, *Stranger to Europe: Poems 1939–1949* (Capetown, South Africa: A.A. Balkema, 1952).

7: NOT GETTING BETTER

104 *Congress, in an attempt to cut costs*: Phone interview with Mark Kander, Director of Health Care Regulatory Analysis for American Speech-Language-Hearing Association, May 31, 2012.

104 *To settle a class-action lawsuit*: Robert Pear, "Settlement Eases Rules for Some Medicare Patients," *New York Times*, October 22, 2012.

8: DHARMA SISTERS

108 *cost between $150 and $200*: "Alzheimer's Drugs: Summary of Recommendations," *Consumer Reports*, accessed September 29, 2011, http://www.consumerreports.org/health/best-buy-drugs/alzheimers.htm.

108 *$2 billion in annual sales*: Katie Thomas, "Drug Dosage Was Approved Despite Warning," *New York Times*, March 23, 2012, B1–B2.

108 *something is being done*: Jane Gross, *A Bittersweet Season* (New York: Random House, 2011), 159.

116 *what Adrienne Rich called*: Adrienne Rich, *Of Woman Born: Motherhood as Experience and Institution* (New York: W. W. Norton, 1995), 236.

125 *One day, two of Bowlby's successors*: Mary Main and Judith Solomon, "Discovery of an Insecure-Disorganized/Disoriented Attachment Pat-

tern," in *Affective Development in Infancy,* ed. Berry T. Brazelton and Michael W. Yogman (Westport, CT: Ablex Publishing, 1986), 95–124.

129 *The path into the light seems dark:* Stephen Mitchell, trans., *Tao Te Ching* (New York: HarperPerennial, 1988), 47.

9: BROKE-DOWN PALACE

131 *astonishingly early age of twenty-two:* David H. Schroeder and Timothy A. Salthouse, "Age Related Effects on Cognition between 20 and 50 Years of Age," *Personality and Individual Differences* 35 (2004): 393–404.

131 *fall by up to 1 percent:* Interview with Timothy Salthouse, Department of Psychology, University of Virginia, Charlottesville, September 10, 2012.

131 *Great breakthroughs in fields such as chemistry:* Timothy Salthouse, "Consequences of Age-Related Cognitive Declines," *Annual Review of Psychology* 63 (2012): 201–226, 211.

131 *Myelin, the fatty white protective sheath:* John H. Morrison and Patrick R. Hof, "Life and Death of Neurons in the Aging Brain," *Science* 278 (1997): 412–16.

132 *10 to 30 percent:* J. Bischkopf, et al., "Mild Cognitive Impairment—A Review of Prevalence, Incidence and Outcome According to Current Approaches," *Acta Psychiatrica Scandinavica* 106, no. 6 (2002): 403–414.

133 *The eye of even a healthy sixty-year-old:* Atul Gawande, "The Way We Age Now," *New Yorker,* April 30, 2007, 50–59.

134 *Some cells undergo destructive metabolic processes:* Steven Austad, *Why We Age* (New York: John Wiley & Sons, 1997), 134.

134 *The ends of our cellular DNA:* Leonard Hayflick, *How and Why We Age* (New York: Ballantine, 1994), 135.

134 *What we call aging is the cumulative effect:* Austad, *Why We Age,* 8, 52–69, 123–45.

134 *more than seven thousand separate degenerative:* Interview with Steven Austad, September 21, 2011.

135 *Many doctors continued to use the cheaper Avastin:* Andrew Pollack, "Cheaper Drug to Treat Eye Disease Is Effective," *New York Times,* April 28, 2011.

138 *Given how much is unknown:* "Risk Factors for Dementia and Cognitive Decline," Source Document, National Health Service of Scotland, October 2003, accessed September 29, 2011, http://www.healthscotland.com/uploads/documents/dementia_LR.pdf.

139 *Half a billion federal dollars:* "Alzheimer's Association—Boomer's Report," Alzheimer's Association, accessed September 29, 2011, http://www.alz.org/boomers.

140 *longevity is the biggest risk factor:* "Alzheimer's Association—Boomer's Report."

140 *only 9 percent*: "Health and Retirement Study," University of Michigan Institute for Social Research and U.S. National Institute on Aging, published in *Alzheimer's & Dementia*, http://www.alzheimersanddementia.org/; cited in Marsha King, "U.S. Dementia Rates Are on the Decline—Memory Loss Isn't Inevitable," *Seattle Times*, February 21, 2008, accessed September 26, 2011, http://seattletimes.com/html/health/2004193111_dementia21m.html.

140 *more than 41 percent*: Maria M. Corrada, et al., "Dementia Incidence Continues to Increase with Age in the Oldest Old: The 90+ Study," *Annals of Neurology* 67 (2010): 114–21.

140 *only one in two hundred*: Benedict Carey, "At the Bridge Table, Clues to a Lucid Old Age," *New York Times*, May 21, 2009, accessed September 30, 2011, http://www.nytimes.com/2009/05/22/health/research/22brain.html?pagewanted=all.

140 *Except their homes*: Judith Graham, "It Comes as a Shock" *New York Times*, Science Times section, September 25, 2012, D7.

142 *When a fine old carpet is eaten by mice*: Jane Hirshfield, *Come Thief* (New York: Alfred A. Knopf, 2011), 19.

142 *like Tintern Abbey*: "Enchanting Ruin: Tintern Abbey and Romantic Tourism in Wales—Romanticism and Ruins," University of Michigan, accessed August 30, 2011, http://www.lib.umich.edu/enchanting-ruin-tintern-abbey-romantic-tourism-wales/ruins.html.

10: WHITE WATER

145 *We lost the mother that we once knew*: Pauline Boss, *Ambiguous Loss: Learning to Live with Unresolved Grief* (Cambridge, MA: Harvard University Press, 2000), 17.

146 *Yale–New Haven was ranked among the top 3 percent*: "Yale–New Haven Hospital Profile," *U.S. News & World Report*, accessed September 14, 2012, http://health.usnews.com/best-hospitals/yale-new-haven-hospital-6160400.

146 *Middlesex Memorial Hospital was rated the safest*: "How Safe Is Your Hospital?" *Consumer Reports*, August 2012, accessed September 25, 2012, http://www.consumerreports.org/cro/magazine/2012/08/how-safe-is-your-hospital/index.htm.

147 *bodily repair services*: Bart Windrum, *Notes from the Waiting Room: Managing a Loved One's End-of-Life Hospitalization* (Boulder, CO: Axiom Action, 2008), 20.

147 *Of those who suffer hospital delirium*: Statistics from the American Geriatrics Society and Sharon Inouye, MD, of Harvard Medical School, cited in Pam Belluck, "Hallucinations in Hospital Pose Risk to Elderly," *New York Times*, June 20, 2010, accessed September 25, 2012, http://www.nytimes.com/2010/06/21/science/21delirium.html.

148 *A Korean folk saying holds:* Pam Belluck, "The Vanishing Mind: Children Ease Alzheimer's in Land of Aging," *New York Times,* November 25, 2010, accessed September 25, 2012, http://www.nytimes.com/2010/11/26/health/26alzheimers.html?pagewanted=all.

11: THE SORCERER'S APPRENTICE

156 *especially, but not only, African-American families:* Melvin Echols Peterson, et al., "Differences in Level of Care at the End of Life According to Race," *American Journal of Critical Care* 19 (2010): 335–43.

156 *a local district attorney might even consider charges:* Lewis M. Cohen, *No Good Deed: A Story of Medicine, Murder Accusations, and the Debate over How We Die* (New York: HarperCollins, 2010).

159 *These devices are seen as simple and low-tech:* Interview with Katrina Bramstedt, January 2007.

160 *They were often deactivated:* Paul S. Mueller, et al., "Deactivating Implanted Cardiac Devices in Terminally Ill Patients: Practices and Attitudes." *Pacing and Clinical Electrophysiology* 31, no. 5 (2008): 560–68.

12: THE BUSINESS OF LIFESAVING

My primary source for the explosion of "Medical Alley" and its subsequent scandals was Kirk Jeffrey, *Machines in Our Hearts: The Cardiac Pacemaker, the Implantable Defibrillator, and American Health Care* (Baltimore: Johns Hopkins University Press, 2001); supplemented by oral interviews with the early movers and shakers (many conducted by Jeffrey) for the Minnesota Oral History Project.

166 *The atmosphere in what would later be nicknamed "Medical Alley":* Kirk Jeffrey, Interview with Anthony J. Adducci, "Pioneers of the Medical Device Industry in Minnesota Oral History Project," Minnesota Historical Society, Roseville, Minnesota, August 9, 2000, 15–28.

167 *Its pacemaker was barely more than a prototype:* David Rhees, interview with Manuel Villafaña, "Pioneers of the Medical Device Industry in Minnesota Oral History Project," Minnesota Historical Society, Plymouth, Minnesota, January and May, 1998, 35.

168 *Spin-offs begat spin-offs:* Kirk Jeffrey, interview with Anthony J. Adducci, 20.

168 *a major advance:* Stephen Westaby with Cecil Bosher, *Landmarks in Cardiac Surgery* (Oxford: Oxford University Press, 1998), 155.

168 *The St. Jude valve became the most commonly used:* James Fogerty, *Con-*

verzatione with Manuel Villafaña, "Pioneers of the Medical Device Industry in Minnesota Oral History Project," Minnesota Historical Society, St. Paul, Minnesota, November 20, 1997, 70.

168 *a handful of pacemaker companies*: David Rhees, interview with Ronald A. Matricaria, "Pioneers of the Medical Device Industry in Minnesota Oral History Project," Minnesota Historical Society, Little Canada, Minnesota, April 21, 2000.

170 *doctors' average incomes quintupled*: Sandeep Jauhar, "Out of Camelot, Knights in White Coats Lose Way," *New York Times,* January 31, 2011, accessed September 17, 2012, http://www.nytimes.com/2011/02/01/health/01essay.html.

170 *Doctors flocked to where the money was*: Paul Starr, *The Social Transformation of American Medicine* (New York: Basic Books, 1982), 359–60.

171 *In all my twenty years experience*: Testimony of Howard F. Hefferman at hearing before the Senate Special Committee on Aging, September 10, 1982. *Fraud, Waste and Abuse in the Medicare Pacemaker Industry,* 31. Transcript reprinted from the collection of the University of Michigan Library. HP. Lexington, Ky. 2012

171 *several executives of Siemens-Pacesetter*: Jeffrey, *Machines in Our Hearts,* 200–201.

172 *At a cardiology conference in Manhattan*: Henry Greenberg, "In Praise of Sudden Death," *Annals of the New York Academy of Science* 382 (1982): 181–82.

172 *Over the next five years*: James S. Todd, Letter to Editor, "Do Practice Guidelines Guide Practice?" *New England Journal of Medicine* 322 (1990): 1822–23.

173 *By 1987, the median income*: Arthur Owens, "How Much Did Your Earnings Grow Last Year?" *Medical Economics,* September 5, 1988, 161.

173 *One of pacemaking's pioneers*: Interview with cardiac surgeon who spoke on condition of anonymity. June 2011.

174 *medical device companies were enjoying*: Centers for Medicare and Medicaid Service, "Health Care Industry Market Update," December 5, 2003; cited in Reed Abelson, "Possible Conflicts for Doctors Are Seen on Medical Devices," *New York Times,* September 22, 2005, accessed September 25, 2012, http://www.nytimes.com/2005/09/22/business/22devices.html?fta=y.

174 *Device-related heart surgeries alone*: "CABG DRG Counts, 2003 CY 100% MEDPAR Short-Stay Files," Centers for Medicare and Medicaid Services. The total represents my computation; it is for cardiac surgeries involving devices only.

174 *$170 billion global industry*: "The North America Medical Instruments & Equipment Sectors: A Company and Industry Analysis," (2004), Mergent, 8–14, accessed July 15, 2011, http://webreports.mergent.com.

174 *Weinstein's "top pick"*: Kenneth N. Gilpin, "MARKET INSIGHT; Is It a Drug Or a Device? Nowadays, Maybe Both," *New York Times,*

May 25, 2003, accessed December 12, 2012, http://www.nytimes
.com/2003/05/25/business/market-insight-is-it-a-drug-or-a-device-now
adays-maybe-both.html.

174 *yet another change in the formulas*: Robert Pear, "White House Alters
Plan to Make Large Cuts in Hospitals' Medicare Payments," *New York
Times,* August 3, 2006, accessed September 25, 2012, http://www
.nytimes.com/2006/08/03/washington/03medicare.html.

175 *AdvaMed hired two former health care staffers*: P. B., "Lobby Shops,"
National Journal, 22 April 2006, accessed via LexisNexis.

175 *inside the Beltway advertising*: Stephen J. Ubl, "AdvaMed: Ensuring
Medical Innovation for All," Medmarc, accessed June 20, 2011, http://
www.medmarc.com/Life-Sciences-News-and-Resources/Articles/Pages/
Ensuring-Medical-Innovation-for-All.aspx#.

175 *spent at least $27 million on lobbying*: "OpenSecrets Lobbying Data-
base," Center for Responsive Politics, accessed June 24, 2012, http://
www.opensecrets.org/lobby/index.php.

175 *They contributed another $1.5 million*: Medical supplies manufac-
turing and sales 2006 campaign contributions, MapLight, accessed
June 22, 2012, http://maplight.org/us-congress/contributions?s=1&
start=01%2F01%2F2006&end=12%2F31%2F2006&office_party=
Senate%2CHouse%2CDemocrat%2CRepublican%2CIndependent
&election=2004%2C2006%2C2008%2C2010%2C2012&business_
sector=Health&business_industry=Pharmaceuticals%2FHealth%20
Products&business_id=H4100&source=All.

175 *After two hundred members of the House and Senate*: Pear, "White House
Alters Plan."

176 *in the estimation of AdvaMed*: Ubl, "AdvaMed."

176 *sham fees*: All of Donigian's charges can be found in United States *ex rel.*
Charles Donigian v. St. Jude Medical, Inc. (D. Mass. January 19, 2010),
Third Amended False Claims Act Complaint, 17, 18, 28, 32–33.

177 *Donigian received $2.6 million*: "Minnesota-Based St. Jude Medical
Pays U.S. $16 Million to Settle Claims that Company Paid Kickbacks
to Physicians," U.S. Department of Justice News Release, January 20,
2011.

177 *The Code of Business Conduct on the St. Jude Web site*: "Code of Business
Conduct," St. Jude Medical, accessed December 12, 2012, available at
Code of Business Conduct page at http://www.sjm.com/.

178 *recused from voting*: "ACC/AHA/HRS 2008 Guidelines for Device-Based
Therapy of Cardiac Rhythm Abnormalities: A Report of the American
College of Cardiology/American Heart Association Task Force on Practi-
cal Guidelines," *Circulation* 117 (May 15, 2008): e405–e6.

179 *nearly a third of its $16.8 million*: "Heart Rhythm Society & Founda-
tion FY11 Revenues from External Sources," Heart Rhythm Society,
accessed April 19, 2012, available at http://www.hrsonline.org/. I followed groundbreaking investigative reporting by ProPublica: Charles

Orenstein and Tracy Weber, "Financial Ties Bind Medical Societies to Drug and Device Makers," *USA Today*, May 5, 2011.

179 *It employed about thirteen hundred sales representatives*: United States *rel.* Charles Donigian v. St. Jude Medical Inc.

179 *and was a member*: "Fortune 500: St. Jude Medical Snapshot," CNNMoney, accessed September 25, 2012, http://money.cnn.com/magazines/fortune/fortune500/2011/snapshots/10595.html.

13: DEACTIVATION

182 *dementia's seven roughly sequential stages*: Susan J. Mitchell, "A 93-Year-Old Man with Advanced Dementia and Eating Problems," *Journal of the American Medical Association* 21, no. 298 (2007): 2527–36.

187 *5 to 10 percent*: Center for Excellence on Elder Abuse and Neglect, University of California at Irvine, "Research Brief: Facts You Need to Know," National Center on Elder Abuse, February 2012.

187 *some griefs augment the heart*: Jane Hirshfield, "Stone and Knife," in *American Poetry Review* 38, no. 5 (September/October 2009), http://www.aprweb.org/issue/septemberoctober-2009.

188 *Ohio State University released a study of the DNA*: Amanda K. Damjanovic, et al., "Accelerated Telomere Erosion Is Associated with a Declining Immune Function of Caregivers of Alzheimer's Disease Patients," *Journal of Immunology* 179, no. 6 (2007): 4249–54.

193 *In a case Bramstedt reported in 2003*: K. A. Bramstedt, "Ethics in Medicine: Questioning the Decision-Making Capacity of Surrogates," *Internal Medicine Journal* 33, nos. 5–6 (2003): 257–59.

195 *beeping and squealing monitors*: Sherwin Nuland, *How We Die* (New York: Vintage Books, 1994), 254.

196 *would not honor his paper DNR*: The only proof of a valid DNR that is reliably honored by paramedics in numerous states is a bracelet from MedicAlert Foundation. See, for example, DNR regulations guidance listed at http://www.ctacep.org (Connecticut). See also "Resources."

197 *recover well enough*: From a 2010 study of more than ninety-five thousand cases of CPR, cited in Ken Murray, "Why Doctors Die Differently," *Wall Street Journal*, February 25, 2012. Adapted from an article first published online in Zocalo Public Square.

14: THE ART OF DYING

212 *did seem to be praising the Lord*: Anthony Froude, *Short Studies on Great Subjects* (London: Longmans, 1884), 2: 99; cited in Frances Comper, ed., *The Book of the Craft of Dying and Other Early English Tracts Concerning Death* (London: Longmans, Green, and Co., 1917), xx.

214 *I forgive you. Good-bye*: Ira Byock, *Dying Well: Peace and Possibilities at the End of Life* (New York: Riverhead Books, 1997), 140. Similar phrasing is used in modern versions of *Ho'oponopono*, the native Hawaiian tradition of forgiveness and reconciliation.

218 *In a study of Zen funeral rituals*: William M. Bodiford, "Zen in the Art of Funerals: Ritual Salvation in Japanese Buddhism," *History of Religions*, Vol. 32, No. 2 (Nov., 1992): 146–64.

15: AFTERWARD

223 *Dying, death, and mourning*: Letters of Eliza Butler, Butler family papers, Corey Library, Rhodes University, Grahamstown, South Africa.

224 *It was a sad noise to hear*: Samuel Pepys, *The Diary of Samuel Pepys*, ed. Henry B. Wheatley (London: George Bell & Sons, 1893), entries for July 30, 1665, and August 31, 1665, available in an online edition, accessed July 25, 2012, http://www.pepysdiary.com/.

229 *white ashes*: Rennyo:16 (Hakotsu no Gobunsho.) *Letters in the Five Fascicle Collection (Gojo Gobunsho)* in *Shinshu Shogyo Zensho*, Vol 3. (Kyoto: Oyagi Kobundo, 1941), 513–14. Translated into English by Hisao Nagaki.

16: VALERIE MAKES UP HER MIND

238 *nearly three billion times*: Arthur E. Weyman and Marielle Scherrer-Crosbie, "Marfan Syndrome and Mitral Valve Prolapse," *Journal of Clinical Investigation*, 114, no. 11 (2004): 1543–46.

239 *He had retired from surgical practice*: The description of Moore's final years is drawn from Atul Gawande's extensive profile, "Desperate Measures," *New Yorker*, May 5, 2003, 70–81.

239 *Losing the Memory*: Sandeep Jauhar, "Saving the Heart Can Sometimes Mean Losing the Memory," *New York Times*, September 19, 2000, accessed September 26, 2012, http://www.nytimes.com/2000/09/19/science/saving-the-heart-can-sometimes-mean-losing-the-memory.html?pagewanted=all&src=pm.

NOTES

17: OLD PLUM TREE BENT AND GNARLED

246 *$80,000 to $150,000*: Estimate, cardiology reimbursement expert Rebecca Sanzone, St. Agnes Hospital, Baltimore, MD. Also data from Medicare listing the median (50th percentile) payments to hospitals for the relevant procedures in 2009. Reimbursements vary widely by region and complications encountered.

246 *a fifth die in intensive care*: Alvin C. Kwok, et al., "The Intensity and Variation of Surgical Care at the End of Life: a Retrospective Cohort Study," *Lancet* 378, no. 9800 (2011): 1408–13.

246 *Medical overtreatment*: Donald M. Berwick and Andrew D. Hackbarth, "Eliminating Waste in US Health Care," *Journal of the American Medical Association*, 307, no. 14 (2012): 1513–16.

246 *13 percent of patients*: K. P. Alexander, et al., "Outcomes of Cardiac Surgery in Patients Aged >/= 80 Years (Results from the National Cardiovascular Network)," *Journal of the American College of Cardiology* 35 (2000): 731–38; cited in Jonathan E. E. Yager and Eric O. Peterson, "Cardiac Surgery in Octogenarians: Have We Gone Too Far or Not Far Enough?" *American Heart Journal* 1147, no. 2 (2004): 187–89.

246 *In a smaller, confirming study*: Mohamed Y. Rady and Daniel J. Johnson, "Cardiac Surgery for Octogenarians: Is It an Informed Decision?" *American Heart Journal* 147, no. 2 (2004): 347–53.

247 *Old plum tree bent*: Eihei Dogen, "Plum Blossoms" (Japanese: "Baika"), *Moon in a Dewdrop,* ed. Kazuaki Tanahashi (San Francisco: San Francisco Zen Center, 1985), 114.

249 *best season of your life*: Wu-men Hui-kai, "Case 19," *The Gateless Gate* (Chinese: *Wu-men kuan*; Japanese: *Mumonkan*). Stephen Mitchell, trans., *The Enlightened Heart: An Anthology of Sacred Poetry* (New York: HarperPerennial, 1993), 47.

20: NOTES FOR A NEW ART OF DYING

282 *lung cancer patients*: J. S. Temel, et al., "Early Palliative Care for Patients with Metastatic Non-Small-Cell Lung Cancer," *New England Journal of Medicine* 353 (2010): 733–42.

BIBLIOGRAPHY

Aoki, Shinmon. *Coffinman*. Anaheim, CA: Buddhist Education Center, 1993.

Ariés, Philippe. *The Hour of Our Death*. Translated by Helen Weaver. New York: Alfred A. Knopf, Inc., 1981.

———. *Western Attitudes Toward Death from the Middle Ages to the Present*. Translated by Patricia M. Ranum. Baltimore: The Johns Hopkins University Press, 1974.

Austad, Steven N. *Why We Age: What Science Is Discovering About the Body's Journey through Life*. New York: John Wiley & Sons, Inc., 1997.

Bailey, Elizabeth. *The Patient's Checklist*. New York: Sterling, 2011.

Bakken, Earl E. *One Man's Full Life*. Medtronic, 1999.

Beaty, Nancy Lee. *The Craft of Dying: The Literary Tradition of* Ars Moriendi *in England*. New Haven, CT: Yale University Press, 1970.

Bennett, Amanda. *The Cost of Hope*. New York: Random House, 2012.

Bevan, Joseph Gurney. *Piety Promoted: In Brief Memorials and Dying Expressions of Some of the Society of Friends, Commonly Called Quakers*. London, United Kingdom: Darton and Harvey, 1838.

Boss, Pauline. *Ambiguous Loss: Learning to Live with Unresolved Grief*. Cambridge, MA: Harvard University Press, 1999.

Brownlee, Shannon. *Overtreated: Why Too Much Medicine is Making Us Sicker and Poorer*. New York: Bloomsbury USA, 2007.

Butler, James, and Jane Garner, eds. *Jim's Journal: The Diary of James Butler*. Johannesburg, South Africa: Witwatersrand University Press, 1996.

Byock, Ira. *The Best Care Possible: A Physician's Quest to Transform Care through the End of Life*. New York: Avery, 2012.

———. *Dying Well: Peace and Possibilities at the End of Life*. New York: Riverhead Books, 1997.

Callahan, Daniel. *Setting Limits: Medical Goals in an Aging Society*. Washington, DC: Georgetown University Press, 2007.

Callahan, Daniel and Angela A. Wasunna. *Medicine and the Market: Equity v. Choice*. Baltimore: The Johns Hopkins University Press, 2006.

Caxton, William, and Heinrich Seuse. *The Book of the Craft of Dying, and Other Early English Tracts Concerning Death*. London, United Kingdom: Longmans, Green, and Co., 1917.

Colby, William H. *Unplugged: Reclaiming Our Right to Die in America*. New York: AMACOM, 2006.

Cooper, David K. C. *Open Heart: The Radical Surgeons Who Revolutionized Medicine*. New York: Kaplan Publishing, 2010.

Devettere, Raymond J. *Practical Decision Making in Health Care Ethics: Cases & Concepts*. Washington, DC: Georgetown University Press, 2000.

Didion, Joan. *The Year of Magical Thinking*. New York: Vintage Books, 2005.

Dormandy, Thomas. *The White Death: A History of Tuberculosis*. New York: New York University Press, 1999.

Dunn, Hank. *Hard Choices for Loving People*. Lansdowne, VA: A & A Publishers Inc., 2009.

Elliot, Carl. *White Coat, Black Hat: Adventures on the Dark Side of Medicine*. Boston: Beacon Press, 2010.

Fadiman, Anne. *The Spirit Catches You and You Fall Down*. New York: Farrar, Straus and Giroux, 1997.

Field, Marilyn J. and Christine K. Cassel, eds. *Approaching Death: Improving Care at the End of Life*. Washington, DC: National Academy Press, 1997.

Foote, Susan Bartlett. *Managing the Medical Arms Race: Innovation and Public Policy in the Medical Device Industry*. Berkeley, CA: University of California Press, 1992.

Foucalt, Michael. *The Birth of the Clinic: An Archaeology of Medical Perception*. New York: Vintage Books, 1994.

Fox, Renne C. *Experiment Perilous: Physicians and Patients Facing the Unknown*. Philadelphia: University of Philadelphia Press, 1959.

Fox, Renee C. and Judith P. Swazey. *The Courage to Fail: A Social View of Organ Transplants and Dialysis*. Chicago: University of Chicago Press, 1973.

Gawande, Atul. *Complications: A Surgeon's Notes on an Imperfect Science*. New York: Picador, 2002.

Glaser, Barney G. and Anselm L. Strauss. *Awareness of Dying*. Chicago: Aldine Publishing Company, 1965.

———. *Time for Dying*. Mill Valley, CA: Sociology Press, 1968.

Greatbatch, Wilson. *The Making of the Pacemaker: Celebrating a Lifesaving Invention*. New York: Prometheus Books, 2000.

Gross, Jane. *A Bittersweet Season: Caring for Our Aging Parents—and Ourselves*. New York: Alfred A. Knopf, 2011.

Gutkind, Lee, ed. *Becoming a Doctor: From Student to Specialist, Doctor-Writers Share Their Experiences*. New York: W. W. Norton & Company, 2010.

Hadler, Nortin M. *Rethinking Aging: Growing Old and Living Well in an Over-treated Society*. Chapel Hill, NC: University of North Carolina Press, 2011.

Hanson, William. *The Edge of Medicine: The Technology That Will Change Our Lives*. New York: Palgrave MacMillan, 2008.

Hall, Stephen S. *Merchants of Immortality: Chasing the Dream of Human Life Extension*. New York: Houghton Mifflin Company, 2003.

Halvorson, George C. and George J. Isham. *Epidemic of Care: A Call for Safer, Better and More Accountable Health Care*. San Francisco: Jossey-Bass, 2003.

Harvey, Peter. *An Introduction to Buddhist Ethics*. Cambridge, United Kingdom: Cambridge University Press, 2000.

Hayflick, Leonard. *How and Why We Age*. New York: Ballantine Books, 1994.

Holck, Frederick H., ed. *Death and Eastern Thought: Understanding Death in Eastern Religions and Philosophies*. New York: Abingdon Press, 1974.

Illich, Ivan. *Medical Nemesis: The Expropriation of Health*. New York: Pantheon Books, 1976.

Jeffrey, Kirk. *Machines in Our Hearts: The Cardiac Pacemaker, the Implantable Defibrillator, and American Health Care*. Baltimore: The Johns Hopkins University Press, 2001.

Jonsen, Albert R. *The Birth of Bioethics*. New York: Oxford University Press, 1998.

Joyce, James. *Dubliners*. New York: Random House, 1954.

Jupp, Peter C. and Clare Gittings. *Death in England*. New Brunswick, NJ: Rutgers University Press, 2000.

Kabat-Zinn, Jon. *Full Catastrophe Living*. New York: Delacorte Press, 1990.

Kalupahana, David J. *Ethics in Early Buddhism*. Honolulu, HI: University of Hawai'i Press, 1995.

Kaufman, Sharon R. *. . . And a Time to Die: How American Hospitals Shape the End of Life*. New York: Scribner, 2005.

Keown, Damien. *Buddhism and Bioethics*. New York: Palgrave, 1995.

Kiernan, Stephen P. *Last Rights: Rescuing the End of Life From the Medical System*. New York: St. Martin's Griffin, 2006.

Lessig, Lawrence. *Republic, Lost: How Money Corrupts Congress—and a Plan to Stop It*. New York: Twelve, 2011.

Lown, Bernard. *The Lost Art of Healing: Practicing Compassion in Medicine*. New York: Ballantine Books, 1996.

Lynn, Joanne. *Sick to Death and Not Going to Take It Anymore!: Reforming Health Care for the Last Years of Life*. Berkeley, CA: University of California Press, 2004.

Lynn, Joanne and Joan Harrold. *Handbook for Mortals: Guidance for People Facing Serious Illness*. New York: Oxford University Press, 1999.

Lynch, Thomas. *The Undertaking: Life Studies from the Dismal Trade.* New York: W. W. Norton & Company, 1997.

Mahar, Maggie. *Money-Driven Medicine: The Real Reason Health Care Costs So Much.* New York: HarperCollins, 2006.

Martensen, Robert. *A Life Worth Living: A Doctor's Reflections on Illness in a High-tech Era.* New York: Farrar, Straus and Giroux, 2008.

McCullough, Dennis. *My Mother, Your Mother: Embracing "Slow Medicine," the Compassionate Approach to Caring for Your Aging Loved Ones.* New York: HarperCollins, 2007.

Miller, G. Wayne. *King of Hearts: The True Story of the Maverick Who Pioneered Open Heart Surgery.* New York: Times Books, 2000.

Moore, Francis D. *Give and Take: The Development of Tissue Transplantation.* New York: Doubleday & Company, 1964.

———. *A Miracle & A Privilege: Recounting a Half Century of Surgical Advance.* Washington, DC: Joseph Henry Press, 1995.

Morris, Charles R. *The Surgeons: Life and Death in a Top Heart Center.* New York: W. W. Norton & Company, Inc., 2007.

Morris, Virginia. *How to Care for Aging Parents.* New York: Workman Publishing, 1996.

Mukherjee, Siddhartha. *The Emperor of All Maladies: A Biography of Cancer.* New York: Scribner, 2010.

Nuland, Sherwin B. *How We Die: Reflections on Life's Final Chapter.* New York: Vintage Books, 1993.

Okun, Barbara and Joseph Nowinski. *Saying Goodbye: How Families Can Find Renewal through Loss.* New York: The Berkeley Publishing Group, 2011.

Peitzman, Steven J. *Dropsy, Dialysis, Transplant.* Baltimore: The Johns Hopkins University Press, 2007.

Pipher, Mary. *Another Country: Navigating the Emotional Terrain of Our Elders.* New York: Riverhead Books, 1999.

Porter, Roy. *The Greatest Benefit to Mankind: A Medical History of Humanity.* New York: W. W. Norton & Company, 1997.

Sogyal, Rinpoche. *The Tibetan Book of Living and Dying.* San Francisco: HarperSanFrancisco, 1994.

Rothman, David J. *Beginnings Count: The Technological Imperative in American Health Care.* New York: Oxford University Press, 1997.

———. *Strangers at the Bedside: A History of How Law and Bioethics Transformed Medical Decision Making.* New York: Basic Books, Inc., 1991.

Safer, Jeanne. *Death Benefits: How Losing a Parent Can Change an Adult's Life—For the Better.* New York: Basic Books, 2008.

Sheehy, Gail. *Passages in Caregiving: Turning Chaos into Confidence.* New York: HarperCollins, 2010.

Starr, Paul. *The Social Transformation of American Medicine.* New York: Basic Books, Inc., 1982.

Tanahashi, Kazuaki, ed. *Moon in a Dewdrop: Writings of Zen Master Dogen.* New York: North Point Press, 1985.

Taylor, Jeremy. *Holy Living and Holy Dying, Volume II: Holy Dying.* Oxford, United Kingdom: Clarendon Press, 1989.

Tilney, Nicholas L. *Invasion of the Body: Revolutions in Surgery.* Cambridge, MA: Harvard University Press, 2011.

Tilney, Nicholas L. *A Perfectly Striking Departure: Surgeons and Surgery at the Peter Bent Brigham Hospital 1912–1980.* Sagamore Beach, MA: Science History Publications, 2006.

———. *Transplant: From Myth to Reality.* New Haven, CT: Yale University Press, 2003.

Van Scoy, Lauren. *Last Wish: Stories to Inspire a Peaceful Passing.* San Diego: Transmedia Books, 2012.

Wanzer, Sidney and Joseph Glenmullen. *To Die Well: Your Right to Comfort, Calm and Choice in the Last Days of Life.* Cambridge, MA: Da Capo Press, 2007.

Welch, H. Gilbert, Lisa M. Schwartz, and Steven Woloshin. *Overdiagnosed: Making People Sick in the Pursuit of Health.* Boston: Beacon Press, 2011.

Windrum, Bart. *Notes from the Waiting Room: Managing a Loved One's End-of-Life Hospitalization.* Boulder, CO: Axiom Action, LLC, 2008.

AUTHOR'S NOTE

I wrote as a reporter and a daughter, and this is a braid of book, part memoir, part medical history, and part investigative journalism. I had full access to my parents' medical and Medicare records and I interviewed many of their doctors. Direct quotations from nonfamily members come from interviews, letters, and medical records and are verbatim, except for minor editing for clarity or rhythm. The names of no doctors have been changed. There are no composite characters, invented quotes, or fabricated scenes.

The family scenes are as accurate as memory, letters, contemporaneous journals, and conversations with surviving family members can make them. Some dialogue is drawn, however, from my fallible memory. I set down events as I remember they occurred, but I may unwittingly have put a few out of chronological order. In a few minor cases, events and chronology described here differ slightly from my account in the *New York Times* article, "What Broke My Father's Heart," due to my discovery of additional letters, journal entries, and other records.

I have taken liberties in describing my inner world. In some places I have included research, memories, or insights that were revealed to me at a later time. In consideration of their privacy, the names of three people—here called Michael, Angela, and Lisa—have been changed, and so have identifying details for members of my mother's support group. The larger truths of the story, I hope, remain intact.

I have not told you everything. But what I have told you is as true as I can make it.

ACKNOWLEDGMENTS

I gratefully acknowledge my debt to those who helped me, both those mentioned here, and many I cannot list by name. You know who you are: thank you for your kindness and generosity.

Brian Donohue, my beloved editor-in-chief, listened to me read almost every chapter of this book aloud, had the integrity to tell me when it was boring, and fed me in every way. My brother Jonathan Butler listened to whole chapters while he drove trucks across country, gave me astute editing suggestions that substantially improved the narrative, and gave me carte blanche to tell my truth. Reporter Nicholas Kusnetz, formerly of ProPublica, found me studies and statistics, fact-checked, and provided crucial investigative reporting on lobbying and the medical device industry. This would not be the book it is without Brian, Jonathan, and Nick.

In New York, I was blessed with expert, dedicated hands.

Thank you to my literary agent, Amanda Urban of International Creative Management, and to Whitney Frick and Nan Graham of Scribner, all of whom provided the kind of editing and care that I'd been told no longer takes place.

Placing our family's medical experience within a wider social context required the help of skilled researchers and fact-checkers, many of them alumni or current students of the University of California's extraordinary graduate school of journalism. Bridget Huber, Rebecca Wolfson, Roberta Kwok, Catherine Traywick, Casey Miner, and Nikki Gloudeman found medical studies and corrected inadvertent errors, working cheerfully and at a high standard. Thank you also to Patrici Flores and Rachel Habib. Book coach Leslie Keenan generously shared with me her mastery of time management, strategic planning, and execution.

Those who read some or all of the manuscript or otherwise provided encouragement and honest feedback (and niggling copyedits) include a posse of old friends, hiking partners, fellow Wesleyan alumni, and fellow writers. Thank you to Elizabeth Andrews, Alison Bartlett, Lisa Bennett, Lauren Cargill, Jonathan Dann, Katherine Ellison, Deirdre English, Mark Fuller, Laura Fraser, Philip Gourevitch, Constance Hale, David Tuller, Jane Hirshfield, and Rachel Houseman.

Thank you also to Barry Jacobs, Elizabeth Krivatsky, Stefanie Marlis, Manijeh Nasrabadi, Barbara Newhouse, Noelle Oxenhandler, Eve Pell, Anna Quindlen, Cathryn Ramin, Catherine Abby Rich, David Roche, Pat Sullivan, Marian Sandmaier, Dani Shapiro, Eva Shoshany, David Sheff, Julia Flynn Siler, Lauren Slater, David Sterry, Jason Roberts, Bart Windrum, Robin Wolaner, and Mel and Patricia Ziegler.

Some passages, in different forms, were previously published in the *New Yorker, Mother Jones, Tricycle, MORE, Psychotherapy Networker,* and the *New York Times Magazine.* Thank you to the editors who helped me to tease out the thinking often half-buried in my first drafts: Charles McGrath, Bernard Ohanian, James Shaheen, Peggy Northrop, Dawn Raffel, Nanette Varian, Rich Simon, Ilena Silverman, and Erica Goode. Thanks also to Rebecca Skloot and her father Floyd for including "What Broke My Father's Heart" in *Best American Science Writing 2011*.

The only way I can fully thank Adam Hochschild, Jack Kornfield, Anne Lamott, Dennis McCullough, Joan Halifax-roshi, Mary Pipher, Sherwin Nuland, and Alexandra Styron for blurbs and early encouragement is to pass on to others the generosity they showed me.

The *New York Times* is a national treasure, and I thank its reporters and contributors Reed Abelson, Pam Belluck, Jane Gross, Anemona Hartocollis, Robin Marantz Henig, Barry Meier, Robert Pear, Tara Parker-Pope, and Paula Span. My debt to the work of Atul Gawande cannot be overstated. His elegantly written fact pieces for the *New Yorker* have helped me, and many others, understand the Rube Goldberg behemoth that is our medical system. For this book, I drew especially on "How We Age Now," "Desperate Measures," "The Cost Conundrum," and "Letting Go." Thanks are due to other writers exploring this forbidden area: first-person pieces by Jonathan Rauch, Michael Wolff, and Sandra Tsing Loh emboldened me. We may not know one another, but we are in conversation. Blue Mountain Center, Hedgebrook Foundation, and Mesa Refuge gave me respite and beautiful, calm places to write and to think during the many years that this book was written and lived.

Scores of scientists, doctors, and academics patiently answered my questions. I wish I could name you all. A few will have to stand for many: Katrina Bramstedt, PhD; S. Andrew Josephson, MD; Rita Redberg, MD; Charles Witherell, MSN,

RN; Victor Parsonnet, MD; and Nicholas Tilney, MD. Numerous doctors at the Mayo Clinic and elsewhere, not listed here by name, gave me an understanding of what "patient-centered medical care" could look like. Ellen Griffith, formerly of the Medicare communications office, was patient, heroic, generous and well-informed, as were her colleagues, Helen Mulligan, Courtney Jenkins, and Kathryn Ceja.

Jeffrey Burns, MD, of Children's Hospital Boston, one of my father's former students, shared his memories of my father and invited me to speak to his first-year students at Harvard Medical School—the opening, I hope, of a continuing national conversation among doctors and families about better shared medical decision making in the last phase of life. Thanks also to Joseph Breault, MD, of Ochsner Clinics in New Orleans, for the privilege of speaking at their inaugural bioethics Grand Rounds.

Gratitude to my dharma sisters and brothers and to the Buddhist teachers who turned and opened my life: Thich Nhat Hanh; Debra Chamberlin-Taylor and Julie Wester of Spirit Rock; and Reb Anderson, Richard Baker, and others at San Francisco Zen Center. I would not be who I am without you.

My late mother, Valerie, entrusted me with her journal to include in the *New York Times* story that formed the foundation for this book and encouraged me, despite her personal inclination toward privacy, to write and publish our family's story. Thank you.

I give thanks to my mother's caregiver's support group, to Ben Carton, Richard Elphick, Diana Wylie, the Rev. M'Ellen Kennedy, and to the Wesleyan community for loving and sustaining my family for decades, and especially to Richard Adelstein for taking my father to lunch.

To those who supported my parents and me during my parents' last eight years: Toni Perez-Palma and Alice Teng, Dr. Robert Fales, and the emergency room, nursing, hospice, and palliative care staffs at Middlesex Memorial Hospital in Middletown, Connecticut, one of the country's finest. A special thanks to the unnamed orderly who gave my father his first poststroke shave. I hope the book makes clear that our family's ordeal resulted from shortcomings in the organization of our medical system, not failings of this excellent hospital.

Readers who responded to my story in the *New York Times Magazine* made me understand that my mother and I were not alone, and there was a need for this book. I especially thank Rachel Houseman, a member of the Facebook group *Slow Medicine*, who e-mailed me to say, "If it helps at 3:00 AM, please know that what you shared made such a huge difference. I learned from you what the picture might likely look like at the end, and because of that, my family was spared the pain that yours endured. . . . I learned from you, and I pass that on to others now." Rachel, believe me, it did help at 3:00 AM.

PERMISSIONS
AND CREDITS

The author wishes to express her thanks to the authors, translators, and license holders of the following books, poems, and photographs for permission to use their copyrighted work. All rights are reserved by the copyright owners for the following:

"I Fell" by Makeda, Queen of Sheba, from *Women in Praise of the Sacred*, edited by Jane Hirshfield (New York: HarperCollins, 1994). Translation © Jane Hirshfield, 1994. Reprinted by kind permission of Jane Hirshfield.

Excerpt from "Plum Blossoms" from *Moon in a Dewdrop* by Dogen, translated by Kazuaki Tanahashi. Translation copyright © 1985 by San Francisco Zen Center. Reprinted by permission of North Point Press, a division of Farrar, Straus and Giroux, LLC.

Excerpt from *Tao Te Ching*, translated by Stephen Mitchell (New York: Harper & Row, 1988). Translation © 1988 by Stephen Mitchell. Reprinted by permission of HarperCollins.

Excerpt from "Ten Thousand Flowers in Spring, the Moon in Autumn" by Wu Men, from *The Enlightened Heart: An Anthology of Sacred Poetry* (New York: HarperPerennial, 1993). Translation © 1993 by Stephen Mitchell. Reprinted by permission of HarperCollins.

Excerpt from "Stone and Knife" from *Come Thief.* © Jane Hirshfield (New York: Knopf, 2011). Reprinted by kind permission of Jane Hirshfield.

Excerpt from "Alzheimer's" from *Come Thief* © Jane Hirshfield (New York: Knopf, 2011). Reprinted by kind permission of Jane Hirshfield.

Excerpt from *Coffinman,* by Shinmon Aoki (English translation of *Nokanfu Nikki*), translated by Wayne S. Yokoyama (Anaheim, CA: Buddhist Education Center, 2002). Translation © 2002 Buddhist Education Center and Wayne S. Yokoyama. All rights reserved. Reprinted by kind permission of Buddhist Education Center.

Excerpt from "To Any Young Soldier" from *Stranger to Europe: Poems 1939–1949* by Guy Butler (Capetown, South Africa: A. A. Balkema, 1952). © 1952 by Guy Butler. Reprinted by kind permission of the Estate of Guy Butler.

PHOTO CREDITS:

Page xii: Photographer Unknown
Page 9: Photograph by Diana Wylie
Page 53: Photograph by Valerie Butler
Page 99: Photograph by Valerie Butler
Page 153: Photograph by Toni Perez-Palma
Page 207: Photograph by Valerie Butler
Page 233: Photograph by Valerie Butler
Page 256: Enso by Valerie Butler
Page 292: Photograph by Toni Perez-Palma